Handbook of Blood Pressure Measurement

Handbook of Blood Pressure Measurement

L. A. Geddes, ME, PhD

Hillenbrand Biomedical Engineering,
Purdue University, West Lafayette, Indiana

Springer Science+Business Media, LLC

Library of Congress Cataloging in Publication Data

Geddes, L. A. (Leslie Alexander), 1921–
Handbook of blood pressure measurement / L. A. Geddes.
p. cm.
Includes bibliographical references and index.
ISBN 978-1-4684-7172-4 ISBN 978-1-4684-7170-0 (eBook)
DOI 10.1007 978-1-4684-7170-0
1. Blood pressure—Measurement—Handbooks, manuals, etc.
I. Title.
[DNLM: 1. Blood Pressure Determination—History. 2. Blood Pressure Determination—instrumentation. 3. Blood Pressure Determination—methods. WG 106 G295h]
QP105.2.G43 1991
612.1'4'0287—dc20
DNLM/DLC
for Library of Congress 90-15638
CIP

Originally published by The Humana Press Inc.,1991
Softcover reprint of the hardcover 1st edition 1991

Preface

During the last two decades, many new techniques and devices have appeared for measuring blood pressure both directly and indirectly. At present, there is no single source for this information; nor is there information on the accuracy and sources of error expected with these technologies. It is for this reason that the present book was written. Divided into three parts: direct measurement, indirect (noninvasive) measurement, and history, the book is directed toward a broad audience in the medical and biological sciences.

Physicians, nurses, medical students, and psychologists, as well as technical persons in the health care field will find Part One of considerable practical value, because it deals with the subject of the accuracy and fidelity of reproduction of blood pressure waveforms that they regularly view on monitors. The definitions of systolic, mean, diastolic, and capillary wedge pressures are illustrated and discussed. The pressures and waveforms at different sites in the cardiovascular system are described in detail. Then the various types of devices for measuring blood pressure are described and thoroughly illustrated. The effect of length and internal diameter of a catheter is analyzed to illustrate how fidelity of reproduction is affected. Simple tests are described that show the reader how to determine the performance characteristics of a catheter–transducer system. The characteristics of catheter-tip transducers are presented, and Part One concludes with a discussion of the rate of change of pressure *(dP/dt)*, what it means, and how such a recording can be calibrated.

Part Two reviews in detail all of the known methods for measuring blood pressure noninvasively. The importance of cuff size, location, body position, and rate of cuff deflation are discussed thoroughly. Then follow descriptions of the palpatory, flush, auscultatory, oscillometric, and ultrasonic methods. The accuracy obtainable with each is presented. Part Two concludes with a discussion of three methods that permit the continuous, noninvasive monitoring of blood pressure.

In the section on history (Part Three), the earliest attempts to measure blood pressure are described, starting with Hales (1733) and progressing to modern disposable, catheter-tip transducers for measuring direct pressure. The second part of the historical account starts with the earliest attempts to measure blood pressure noninvasively.

The evolution of the concept of counterpressure is traced from its beginning to its practical application with the arm-encircling cuff. Also included is a reproduction of Korotoff's paper on the auscultatory method and a translation of it, along with excerpts from his MD thesis that describes how he was led to adopt the auscultatory method.

In 1970 the author published a monograph with a similar title that has been out of print for about a decade. This book and its predecessor derived from lectures to medical students, nurses, clinicians, biomedical engineers, and researchers. In the present updating, every effort has been made to make the material easy to read and use without the need of previous training or special skills.

L. A. Geddes

Contents

Part Three

PART ONE

The Direct Measurement of Blood Pressure

INTRODUCTION

Although Galen (130–200 AD) palpated the pulse and classified it in terms of strength, rate and rhythm, it was not until 1733 when Stephen Hales measured arterial pressure directly in an unanesthetized horse that was cast to the ground. He connected a long vertical glass tube to the femoral (crural) artery (and later to the carotid) and observed the blood to rise 8 ft 3 in. above the level of the left ventricle. He reported cardiac and respiratory variations on the height of the column of blood. The mean pressure corresponding to 99 inches of blood is 186 mm Hg. However, it was not until 1828 when the mercury U-tube manometer was introduced by Poiseuille that we obtained our units for measuring blood pressure (mm Hg). Figure 1 illustrates Poiseuille's manometer.

Systolic and diastolic pressure were first measured accurately by Fick (1864) who employed a Bourdon tube coupled to a stylus that inscribed the record on a smoked-drum kymograph.

SYSTOLIC, MEAN, AND DIASTOLIC PRESSURES

Before proceeding with a discussion of the various devices that measure blood pressure directly, it is worthwhile establishing the meaning of systolic, mean, and diastolic pressures. Figure 2 illustrates a typical aortic pressure record. Systolic is the peak, and diastolic is the minimum pressure. The pulse pressure is the difference between systolic and diastolic pressures. Mean pressure is determined by measuring the area under the pressure curve over

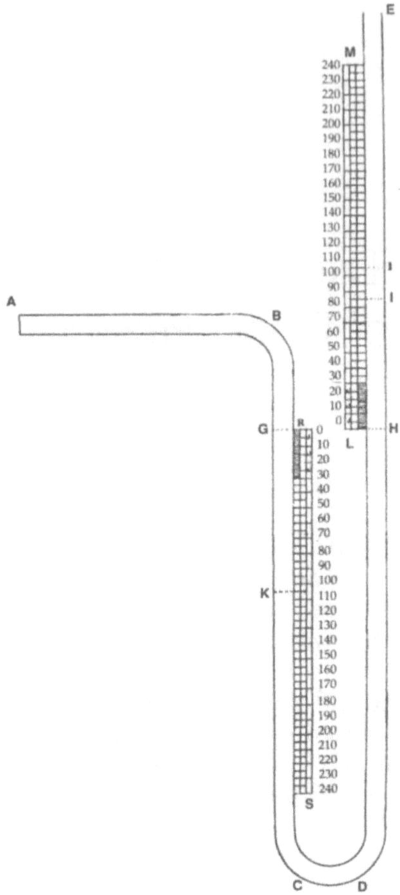

Fig. 1. Poiseuille's mercury U-tube manometer (From Poiseuille, J. L. M., *La Force du Coeur Aortique*. Thesis presented to the Faculty of Medicine, (Univ. Paris), Aug. 8, 1828, for the Doctorate in Medicine.

one cardiac cycle, and dividing this area by the cardiac period, i.e., the base of the measured area, as shown in Fig. 2. Mean pressure is not the average of systolic and diastolic pressures; nor is it diastolic pressure plus one third of pulse pressure. Because the arterial pulse waveform depends on the site selected for measurement, the mean pressure is site dependent. It is possible to state that mean pressure is diastolic pressure plus K times pulse pressure. Because the contour of the pulse wave is different at different sites, K is site dependent. Figure 3 illustrates arterial pressure waveforms at different distances from the aortic valve. Note that the pulse wave becomes

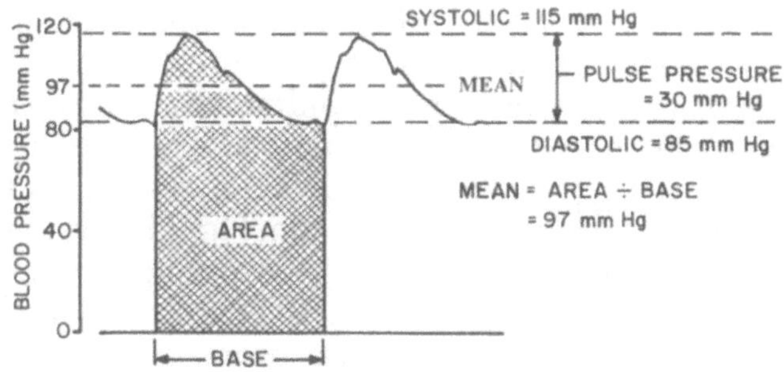

Fig. 2. Systolic, mean, and diastolic pressures.

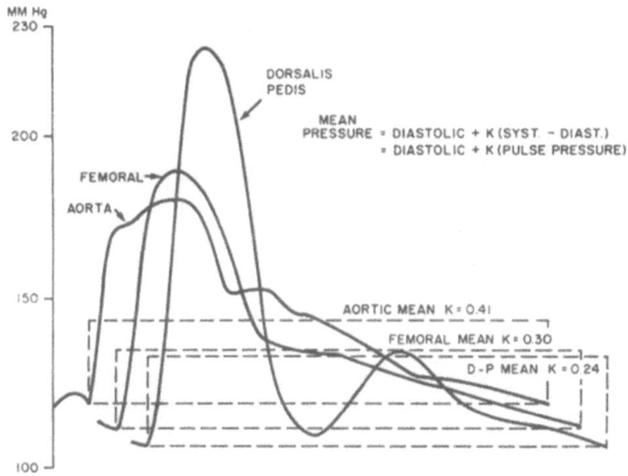

Fig. 3. Pressures at three sites in the arterial system, and the values for K.

peaked with increasing distance from the heart. Thus, the systolic pressure in the femoral and dorsalis pedis arteries, in a recumbent subject, is slightly higher than systolic pressure in the ascending aorta. Diastolic and mean pressures decrease with increasing distance from the aortic valve.

Many attempts have been made to enable calculation of mean pressure ($\overline{P}$) from systolic (S) and diastolic (D) pressures. Unfortunately, this is not possible with accuracy. The following expression is sometimes used:

$$\overline{P} = D + K(S - D)$$

The factor K depends on the site, as shown in Fig. 3. Values from about 0.2 to 0.4 are typical. However, K also depends on blood pressure, as shown by Voelz (1981). This is not surprising because the elasticity of arteries depends on pressure.

The pressure waveform in the pulmonary artery is similar to that in the aorta; however, pulmonary artery pressure is much lower. Figure 4 is a typical record showing a systolic pressure of 26 mm Hg, and a diastolic pressure of 10 mm Hg. The systolic pressure in the right ventricle exceeds that in the pulmonary artery. Likewise, systolic pressure in the left ventricle exceeds that in the aorta. These differences reflect the pressure drops across the pulmonic and aortic valves, respectively. The diastolic pressure in the right and left ventricle ranges from a few to about 10 mm Hg in a normal subject, as shown in Fig. 4.

It is of interest to observe that mean pressure in the aorta is much higher than that in the left ventricle because the aorta is separated from the ventricle by the aortic valve. Figure 5 illustrates respiration and left-ventricular systolic and diastolic pressures (left). During recording of the latter, mean pressure was derived electronically, as shown in Fig. 5. Then, left ventricular systolic and diastolic pressures were displayed; then, the tip of the pressure-recording catheter was pulled into the aorta, revealing aortic systolic and diastolic pressures, following which aortic mean pressure was derived electronically.

In practice, it is highly desirable to know left-ventricular, end-diastolic pressure (LVEDP) because this is the preload for the left ventricle. Increasing preload (up to a point) increases the force of contraction; this phenomenon is known as the Frank-Starling (or Starling's) law, and an example of this is shown in Fig. 6. An excessive preload (LVEDP) can result in a less forceful contraction, and identifies the pressure at which the left ventricle cannot respond, thereby identifying beginning failure of the contractile process.

The accurate measurement of left-ventricular preload requires catheterization of the left ventricle, that is difficult and not without risk. Instead, a catheter can be passed pervenously into the pulmonary artery to obtain an estimate of left-ventricular, end-diastolic pressure. By advancing a balloon-tipped (Swan-Ganz) catheter through the right atrium, ventricle, and far into a small branch of pulmonary artery, it is possible to measure a pressure that is a good estimate of left-ventricular, end-diastolic pressure. The pressure so measured is called pulmonary capillary wedge (PCW) pressure.

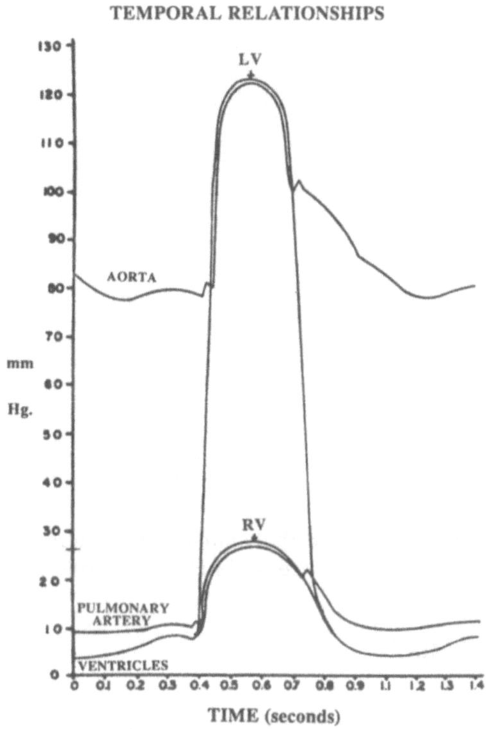

Fig. 4. Right and left-sided pressures. (Redrawn from *Cardiovascular Sound*. V. McKusick, Baltimore, 1958, Williams & Wilkins, 570 pp.)

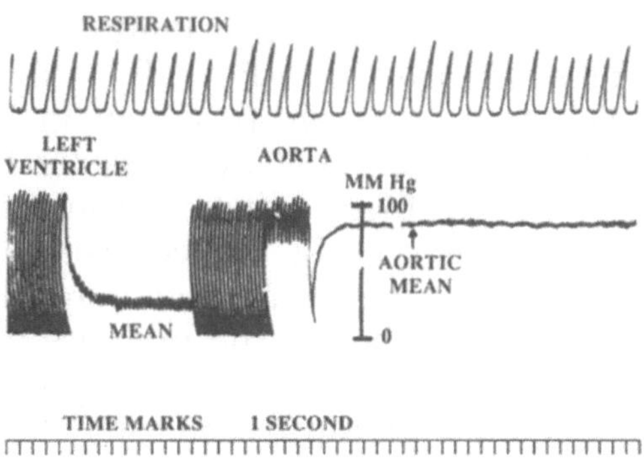

Fig. 5. Systolic, diastolic, and mean left-ventricular pressures, left. On the right, the catheter was pulled back into the aorta to reveal aortic systolic and diastolic pressures and then aortic mean pressure.

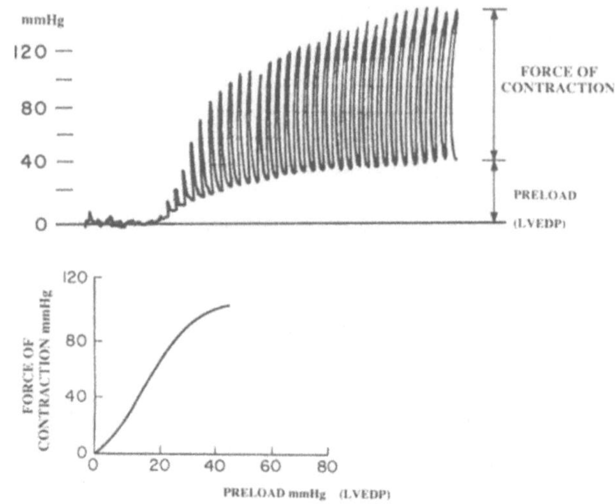

Fig. 6. Starling's law of the heart that states that an increase in diastolic pressure (preload or LVEDP) results in an increased force of contraction. (Illustration courtesy of M. Niebauer.)

WEDGE PRESSURE

The concept of wedge pressure can best be understood by first considering blood flow (Q) along a uniform vessel. Such a case is shown in Fig. 7, and the pressure drop ($P_1 - P_2$) is defined by Poiseuille's law, which states that the flow (Q) is proportional to the pressure drop ($P_1 - P_2$), the geometry of the vessel (radius r, length L), and the viscosity (n) of the blood. If there is no flow ($Q = 0$), there will be no pressure drop, i.e., $P_1 - P_2 = 0$.

A catheter placed in a vessel, as shown in Fig. 8, will not measure the pressure in organ A. Now consider the situation in which a pressure-sensing catheter is wedged into a branch of the pulmonary artery, as shown in Fig. 9. Because the catheter tip is wedged in the vessel, flow is arrested; therefore, there will be no pressure drop beyond the catheter. The pressure measured at the catheter tip will be an estimate of left atrial (LA) pressure, and when the mitral valve is open, the pressure is an estimate of left ventricular, end-diastolic pressure (LVEDP). This pressure is designated pulmonary capillary wedge (PCW) pressure.

Pulmonary capillary wedge pressure is measured by floating a balloon-tipped Swan-Ganz catheter (Fig. 10A) into the pulmonary artery while recording pressure from the catheter tip. Figure 10B illustrates a typical pressure record when advancing the catheter

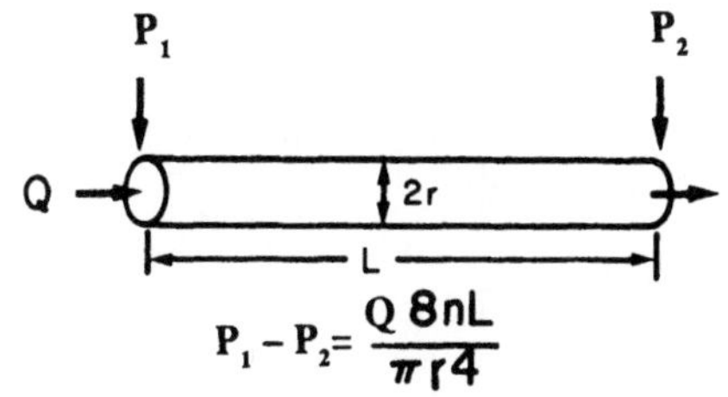

Fig. 7. Poiseulle's Law

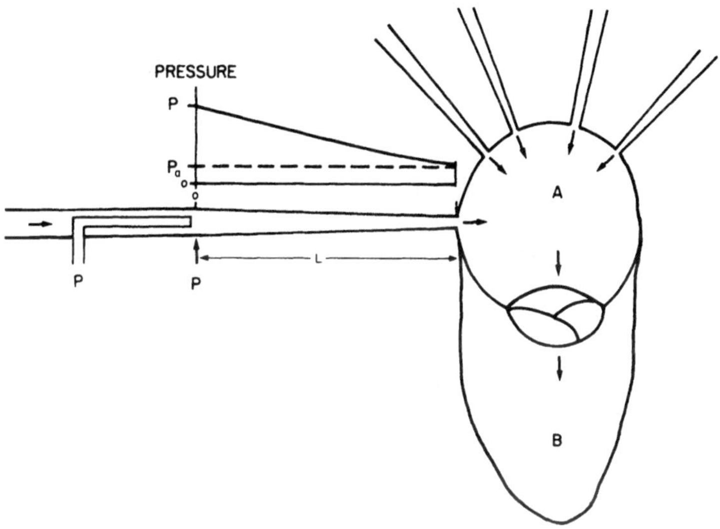

Fig. 8. The pressure drop along one of many vessels entering chamber A.

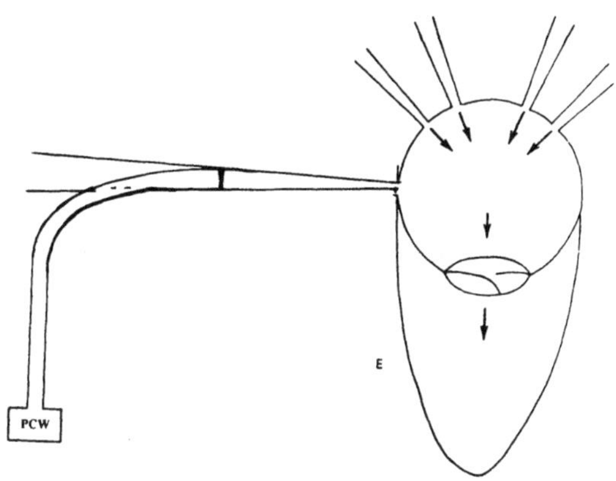

Fig. 9. Catheter used to measure pulmonary capillary wedge (PCW) pressure.

(A)

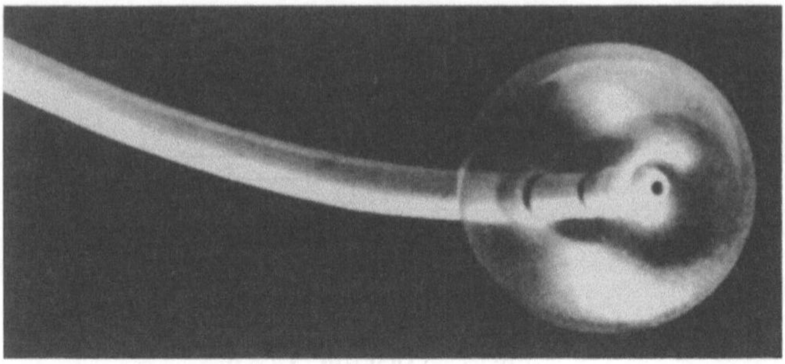

(B)

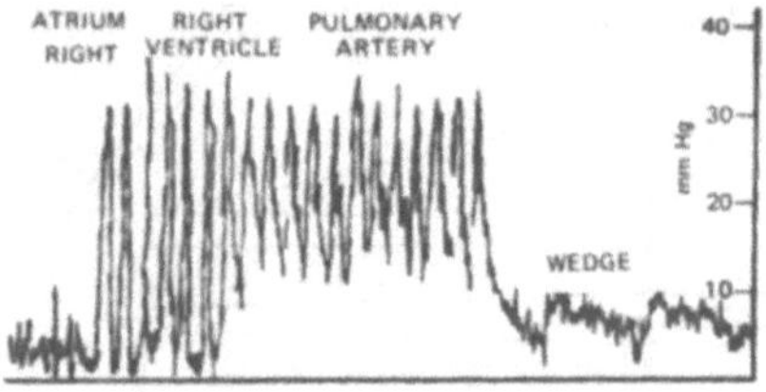

Fig. 10. Swan-Ganz, balloon-tipped catheter (A), and pressure record (B) as the tip is advanced through the right atrium, ventricle, and into the pulmonary artery, then becoming wedged to reveal pulmonary capillary wedge pressure. (Courtesy, Electro-Catheter Corp. Rahway N.J.).

through the right atrium, ventricle, and into the pulmonary artery, and continuing to advance it into the wedged position, as shown in the right of Figure 10B.

VARIATIONS IN BLOOD PRESSURE

Although a well-regulated quantity, blood pressure is not constant; it varies with respiration and heart rate. Moreover, there are vasomotor waves with a frequency of several per min that reflect a striving of the regulatory system to maintain a constant pressure. Figures 11A, B illustrate typical variations in blood pressure with respiration. Figure 11C illustrates vasomotor (Traube-Hering) waves. Observe that the higher frequency respiratory variations can be identified on the low-frequency vasomotor waves. Such waves are often seen with medullary hypoxia, and during prolonged anesthesia.

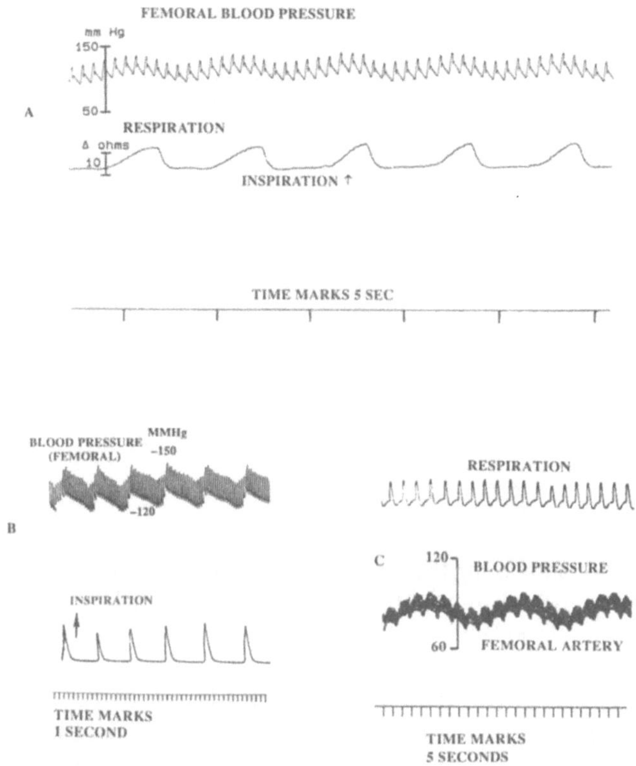

Fig. 11. Respiratory variations in blood pressure (A, B), and vasomotor and respiratory waves (C).

HYDROSTATIC HEAD

Blood pressure is referenced to environmental pressure. However, the site of measurement and the level of the transducer merit special attention. The hydrostatic reference for blood-pressure measurement is the level of the right atrium. If the blood pressure transducer is below this level, the measurement pressure (irrespective of the measurement site), will be falsely high. If the transducer is above the level of the left atrium, the measured pressure will be falsely low. The following experiment clearly demonstrates these facts.

Figure 12A (left) illustrates a blood pressure recording made with the transducer at the level of the left atrium. In Fig. 12A (center), the transducer was lowered 40 cm, and observe the apparent increase in blood pressure. After about 50 s, the transducer was lowered to the level of the left atrium. In Fig. 12B (left), the record-

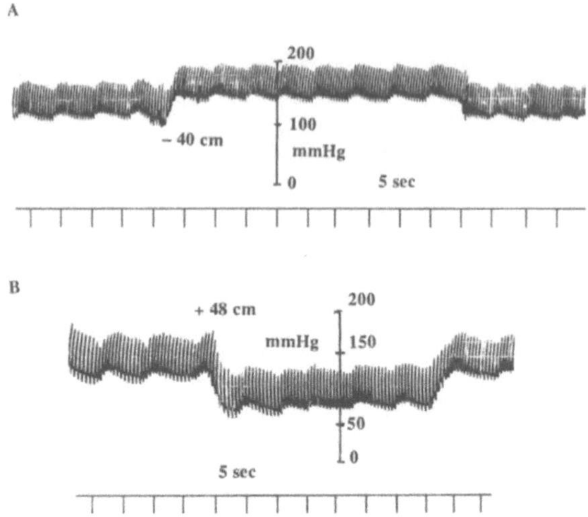

Fig. 12. Effect of lowering the transducer 40 cm (A) and raising the transducer 48 cm (B) from the level of the right atrium. (From Geddes, L. A., *Journ. Clin. Eng.* 1986, **II:** 481–482. By permission.)

ing was made with the transducer at the level of the left atrium. In the center of the figure is the record made by raising the transducer 48 cm above the level of the left atrium. Note the apparent decrease in blood pressure. After 30 s, the transducer was returned to the level of the right atrium, as shown in Fig. 12B, right. It should be pointed out that the use of a long catheter from an artery to the transducer at the level of the right atrium will not provide an error in mean pressure. However, the fidelity of the pulse wave will be distorted, and systolic and diastolic pressure will be in error because pulse pressure will be reduced. This subject is discussed elsewhere in this chapter.

The foregoing clearly demonstrates the importance of locating the transducer at the level of the right atrium. It is of value to be aware of the error that can be introduced by an intervening hydrostatic head. Because pressure transducers and their catheters are filled with saline, that has a density of very nearly 1 gm/mL, it is easy to calculate the equivalent pressure in mm Hg, represented by a fluid column of any height. For example, if a one foot (12 in.) of difference in level exists, the equivalent pressure is $12 \times 25.4 = 304.8$ mm H_2O. The density of mercury is 13.58 gm/mL; therefore, the equivalent pressure of one foot of saline is $304.8/13.58 = 22.4$ mm Hg. It is important to recognize that it is not the length of catheter connected to the transducer that produces the hydrostatic error, it is the difference in level between the transducer and the level of the left atrium.

FREQUENCY CONTENT OF A BLOOD-PRESSURE WAVEFORM

The ability of a catheter-transducer system to produce a signal that is a faithful copy of the blood-pressure presented to the tip of the catheter is described in terms of the hydraulic sinusoidal frequency response. This relationship is expressed as a plot of the ratio of the transducer output (the electrical signal) to the input (the amplitude of sinusoidally varying pressure at different frequencies), vs frequency. It is important to recognize the implications of this relationship. The starting point is to distinguish between frequency and frequency content of a pressure wave. The easiest way to introduce this concept is to recognize that middle C (256 cycles/s) struck on a piano does not sound like a note of the same frequency played on a violin. The reason for the difference is because each has different overtones or harmonics. It is the particular harmonic content that gives a musical note its characteristic quality. A harmonic has a frequency that is a multiple of the fundamental frequency.

Fourier, a French mathematician, showed that any periodic complex wave can be synthesized by a series consisting of a constant (the mean value of the waveform over one cycle), plus an infinite series of cosine and sine waves, the frequencies of which are multiples (harmonics) of the frequency of the complex wave, i.e., the fundamental frequency. Sine and cosine waves are the simplest mathematical waves. Fourier gave the rules for calculating the amplitude of each harmonic. When all of the harmonics are added, the original complex wave is reproduced. In a practical application, often, only sine or cosine wave components are present. Also, it will be seen that the amplitudes of the higher frequency harmonics decrease with increasing harmonic frequency.

It is not necessary to go into the mathematics that underlie computation of the amplitudes and frequencies of each harmonic needed to synthesize a blood-pressure waveform. Instead, a few examples can be given to illustrate the concept of the frequency content of a blood-pressure wave. For example, in Fig. 13A is shown two sine waves of frequency f and 2f, representing the fundamental sine wave (that would correspond to the cardiac frequency f in beats

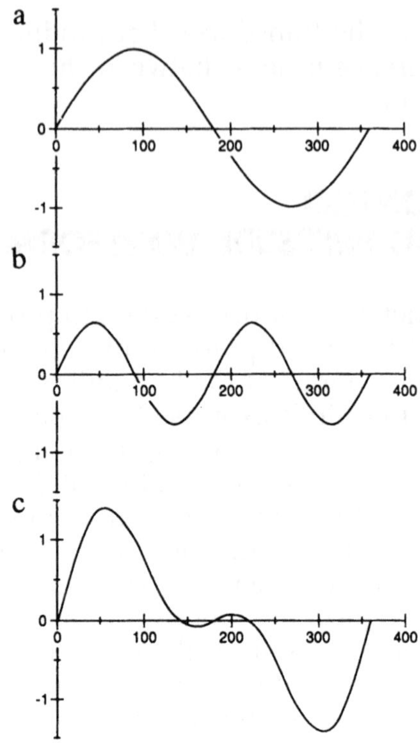

Fig. 13. Summation of the fundamental (A), and 63.2% of the second harmonic (B), to synthesize a blood-pressure wave (C).

per s), and the second harmonic, another sine wave with a frequency of 2f (Fig. 13B). The amplitude of the fundamental is 100%, and that of the second harmonic is 63.2%. Addition of these two components is shown in Fig. 13C, exhibiting a waveform that crudely resembles an arterial pressure wave.

By adding the higher frequency harmonics (with their correct amplitudes specified by the Fourier series), it is possible to obtain an excellent reproduction of a blood-pressure wave. Figure 14A makes this point by adding the amplitudes of the first six harmonics. The dark curve is the original blood-pressure wave; the lighter curve just below it is the reconstruction obtained by summing the instantaneous amplitudes of the first six harmonics. The peak amplitudes of each (in relation to that of the fundamental) are shown in the inset of Fig. 14A. In Fig. 14B are shown the amplitudes of the frequency components for pressure waves measured at various sites in the vascular system.

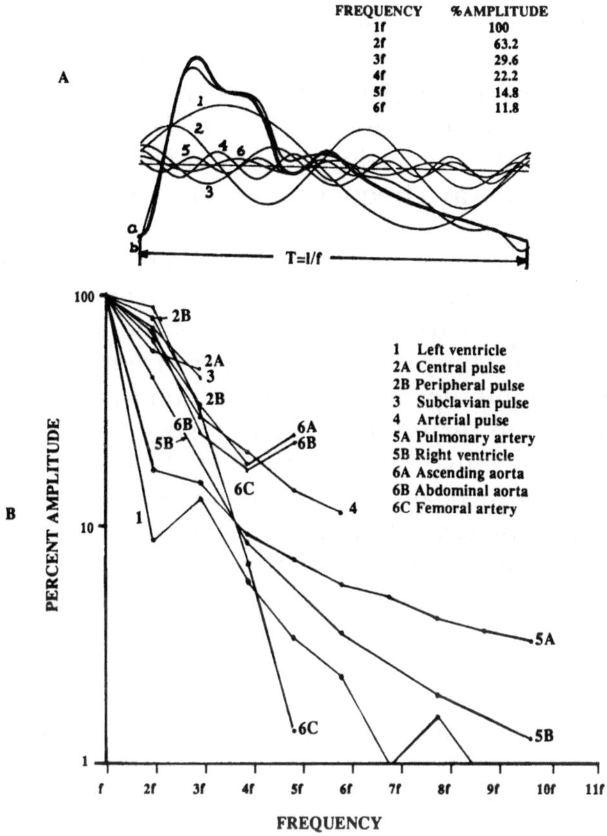

Fig. 14. In A is shown blood pressure waveform (dark curve) and its reproduction by summing the instantaneous amplitudes of the first six harmonics (Redrawn from Hansen, A. T., *Pressure Measurement in the Human Organism,* Copenhagen, 1949, Teknisk Forlag). In B are shown the amplitudes of the harmonics for various blood pressure waveforms (Redrawn from Geddes, L. A., *The Direct and Indirect Measurement of Blood Pressure,* Chicago, 1970, Year Book Publishers Inc.).

It is now possible to bring together the essential facts pertinent to the frequency content of a blood-pressure waveform. For all waveforms, it is clear that the amplitudes of the harmonics decrease with increasing harmonic frequency. It is logical to inquire about the number of harmonics needed for faithful reproduction. The answer is related to the fidelity desired. However, in practice, including at least up to the sixth harmonic provides a good reproduction. Inclusion of up to the tenth harmonic provides very good reproduction. Therefore, for an adequate reproduction of the blood pressure waveform of a subject at rest with a heart rate of 72 beats/min (1.2

beats/s, the fundamental), provision of a uniform sine-wave frequency response extending to $6 \times 1.2 = 7.2$ Hz is adequate. If the subject's heart rate were 180 beats/min, a uniform sine wave frequency response extending to $6 \times 3 = 18$ Hz would be required. If high-fidelity reproduction is desired (i.e., inclusion of up to the 10th harmonic), the sine wave frequency response would need to extend to 30 Hz for the latter case.

It was stated earlier that the Fourier series contained a constant that is the mean value of the waveform over one cycle. When applied to blood pressure, this quantity is the mean pressure. In point of fact, this component is the zero-frequency component. Therefore, for a good reproduction of the blood-pressure waveform, the hydraulic sine wave frequency response of the catheter-transducer system must extend from 0 Hz to six times the highest cardiac frequency in beats per s. A better reproduction would be obtained with a sine wave frequency response extending from 0–10 times the cardiac frequency in beats/s.

In the foregoing discussion, attention was focused on the sine wave frequency response of the catheter-transducer system. In point of fact, the sine wave frequency response required is that from the catheter tip to the display. It is very easy to provide a more-than-adequate frequency response in the electronics from the transducer to the display. If high fidelity reproduction is desired, filters should not be placed in the electronic amplifier-display system.

TYPES OF TRANSDUCERS

Mercury Manometer

Although not a modern blood-pressure transducer, the mercury manometer is important for two reasons

1. It is used to calibrate all blood pressure transducers; and
2. It can be used to measure mean arterial pressure.

Some of the subtleties of this noble instrument will now be presented.

Figure 15A illustrates the mercury-filled U-tube manometer. The application of pressure (P) causes the level of mercury in the left side to fall, and that in the right side to rise, as shown in Fig. 15B.

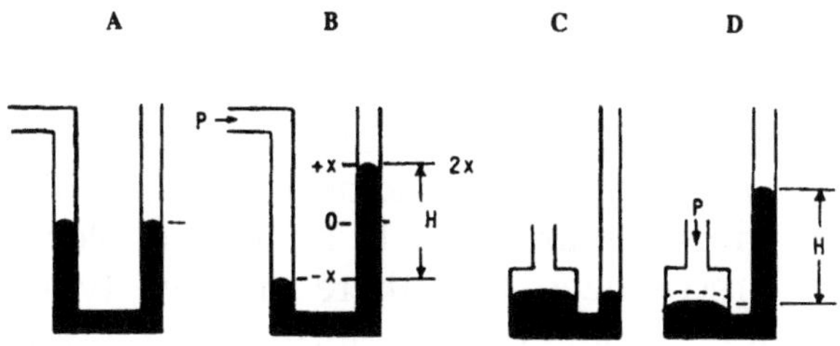

Fig. 15. The mercury manometer. In A is shown a manometer with arms of equal cross-sectional area. In B, the applied pressure (P), causes the mercury in the left tube to fall and that in the right tube to rise; the pressure in mm Hg is H. In C is shown a mercury manometer in which the left tube is larger in diameter than in the right tube. When a pressure P is applied, the mercury in the left tube falls slightly, that in the right tube rises more; the pressure in mm Hg is H (Redrawn from Geddes, L. A., *Cardiovascular Devices*, New York, 1984, John Wiley & Sons).

The pressure in mm Hg is the height (H). Note that the mercury level in the left tube fell x units, and that in the right tube rose x units; the pressure (P) that produced this change is 2× mm Hg. In any mercury manometer, the pressure is the height (H) of the column of mercury that is supported by the pressure.

The mercury manometer used with sphygmomanometers is of the type shown in Fig. 15C. Note that the diameter of the tube on the left is larger than that on the right. The application of a pressure (P) to the left tube causes the mercury to fall slightly therein, and to rise more in the right-hand tube as shown in Fig. 15D. The pressure is the height (H) of the column of mercury.

With the mercury manometer shown in Fig. 15C, the pressure scale is mounted alongside the narrow tube on the right. Because of the unequal areas of the two tubes, one division on the scale is not equal to one millimeter, it is less, the amount depending on the ratio of the areas of the two tubes.

It was stated earlier that the mercury manometer can be used to display mean arterial pressure. By fluid filling the communication (catheter) to the artery and the tubing up to the mercury, the mercury in the left tube will fall, and that in the right tube will rise. Small amplitude oscillations having the cardiac frequency will be evident. The mean height (H) so displayed is true mean arterial pressure. Owing to the large inertia of the mercury column, and viscous damping, the maximum and minimum of the oscillations do not represent systolic and diastolic pressure.

Electrical Transducers

All modern blood-pressure transducers operate on the basis of the electrical detection of the deflection of an elastic member exposed to blood pressure. Although this basic principle underlies their operation, different strategies are used to obtain the electrical signal. It should also be recognized that there are two types of pressure transducer; catheter type, and catheter-tip type. Both types will be described in detail.

Catheter-Type Transducers

At present, there is an increasing number of prepacked, sterilized disposable pressure transducers becoming available. However, many of their predecessors are still in use; therefore, it is desirable to describe the operating principles of all of these types.

Figure 16A illustrates the principle underlying the operation of all catheter-type pressure transducers in which the elastic member that is deflected by pressure is represented as a spring (K)-loaded piston. The applied pressure P(t) causes the piston to move x units, the movement being detected electrically. The back of the piston is vented to environmental (atmospheric) pressure. With the application of pressure, a small volume (Ax) of fluid enters the transducer. Figure 16B illustrates a long catheter connected to the transducer, and blood pressure P(t) is presented to the tip of the catheter.

Strain-Gauge Transducer

The transducer that made blood-pressure recording practical and easy was the Statham strain-gauge unit (Lambert and Wood, 1947) that is illustrated in Fig. 17A. Strain is defined as extension per unit length ($\Delta L/L$). Strain applied to a wire increases its length, and decreases its diameter. Both effects increase its electrical resistance. In the Statham transducer (Fig. 17A), the pressure (P) acting on the corrugated diaphragm causes the block b to move to the right. Affixed to the block are four strain-gauge elements (1–4). The tension in 2 and 3 increases, thereby increasing their resistance; the tension in 1 and 4 decreases, thereby decreasing their resistance. The four strain-gauge elements form a Wheatstone bridge that is unbalanced, and provides an output signal when pressure (P) is

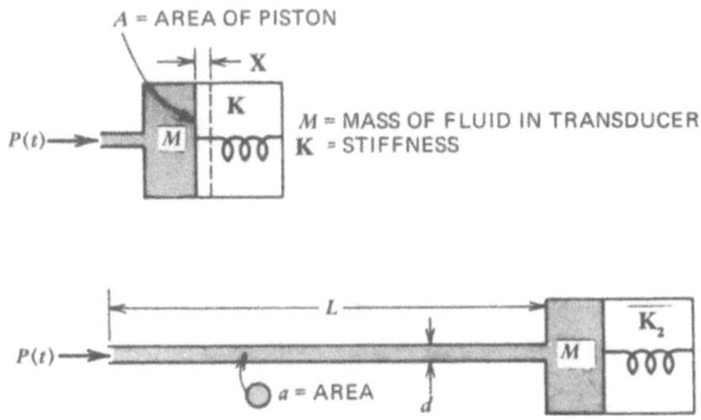

Fig. 16. Principle employed in the catheter-type pressure transducer. The elastic diaphragm has been represented by a piston operating against a spring K. Application of a pressure P(t) causes a small amount of fluid to enter the transducer. Detection of displacement of the diaphragm (i.e., displacement x of the idealized piston) is accomplished electrically to produce a recordable signal.

applied. Because the four active strain-gauge elements are arranged in a bridge circuit, temperature changes affect each element in the same way, and the bridge does not become unbalanced with a temperature change. The output of the Statham (Gould) pressure transducer is typically 5μV per mm Hg of pressure, per volt of excitation. The transducer can accommodate up to about 10 volts for excitation.

Figure 17B illustrates the Bell and Howell strain-gauge pressure transducer. The strain-gauge wires are wrapped around insulated posts mounted at right angles to a spring member in the form of a cross. Pressure applied to the diaphragm is coupled to the cross by the force rod that bends the cross, causing the tension to increase in the wires above the cross, and to decrease in those below. The strain-gauge elements are arranged to form a Wheatstone bridge circuit that provides an output with the application of pressure. This arrangement provides temperature stability. The output is typically 5μV per mm Hg per volt of excitation applied to the transducer.

Disposable Dome

The advent of disposable pressure transducers caused the manufacturers of nondisposable pressure transducers to provide sterilized, disposable domes for their transducers. The dome of a pressure transducer is the top part that is fluid filled (Fig. 16). The disposable

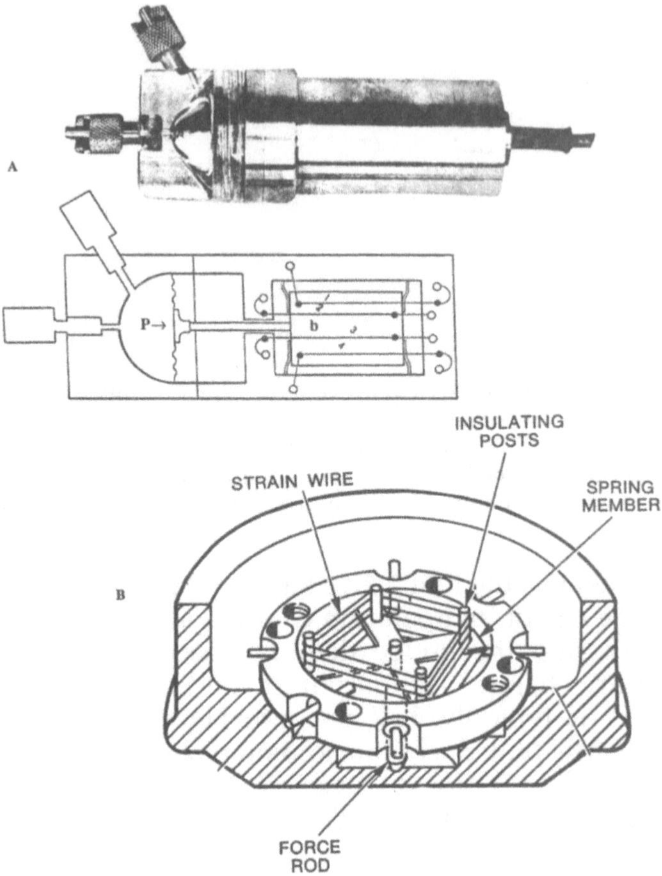

Fig. 17. Strain-gauge transducers. A, Statham (Gould), and B, Bell and Howell.

dome contains a thin compliant membrane (dome diaphragm) that separates the fluid in the catheter and dome from the transducer diaphragm, as shown in Fig. 18. The pressure in the fluid in the dome is communicated to the transducer diaphragm via this membrane. Often, a thin fluid film is employed to minimize the risk of creating an air space between the dome and transducer diaphragm that would increase the volume displacement, and adversely affect the performance of the transducer.

Usually, the membrane in the dome is strong enough to permit unscrewing and removal of the transducer. In this way, a patient can be transported or the transducer replaced. Attractive and practical as such domes are, great care must be exercised to assure that the dome diaphragm communicates evenly with the transducer diaphragm.

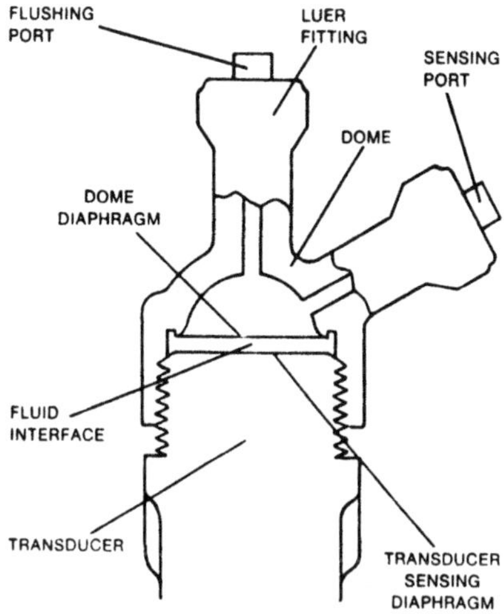

Fig. 18. Disposable, sterilized, interchangeable dome for strain-gauge pressure transducer.

Capacitive Transducer

Two conducting surfaces (e.g., plates), separated by an insulator (dielectric), constitute a capacitor. The capacitance depends on the area of the surfaces, and inversely with their separation. A decrease in separation increases the capacitance that can give rise to an electrical signal.

One manufacturer (Hewlett-Packard) provides a transducer in which the elastic member deflected by blood pressure is a quartz diaphragm coated with a conducting film that forms the moving plate of the capacitor. The other plate of the capacitor is fixed and nearby. Figure 19 illustrates this transducer The circuitry built into the device allows it to be connected to any instrument designed to accommodate conventional strain-gauge transducers.

Disposable Pressure Transducer

Integrated-circuit technology has now made it possible to create high-quality, low-cost, disposable pressure transducers. The first member of this family was introduced by Cobe Laboratories (Denver, CO), and is shown in Fig. 20. Being originally developed for the automotive industry by Microswitch Co. (Freeport, IL), it was reconfigured to permit fluid filling, thereby allowing the measurement of blood pressure.

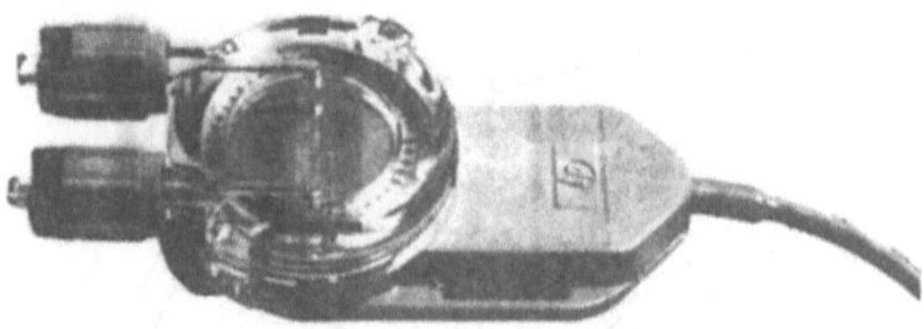

Fig. 19. The Hewlett-Packard capacitive blood-pressure transducer.

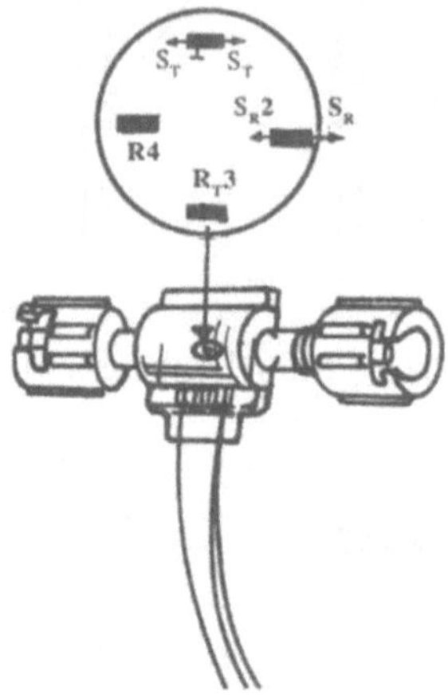

Fig. 20. The Cobe sterilized, disposable pressure transducer. The inset shows the location of the four strain-gauge elements on the back of the diaphragm. (Courtesy, Cobe Lab., Denver, CO and Microswitch, Freeport, IL).

The Cobe sterilized, disposable pressure transducer (Fig. 20) consists of a small silicon diaphragm coated with an insulating compound to prevent corrosion by the fluid in the dome, and to provide electrical insulation. The back of the diaphragm is vented to atmospheric pressure. On the back of the diaphragm (Fig. 20-1234) is deposited the four strain-gauge elements that are arranged in a Wheatstone bridge circuit to provide temperature stability. The output typically 8μV/mm Hg. per volt of excitation applied to the transducer.

DYNAMIC RESPONSE OF BLOOD-PRESSURE TRANSDUCERS

Refer to Figure 16A that displays the transducer modeled as a frictionless piston that acts against a spring of stiffness K. The transducer dome is filled with fluid having a mass M. Therefore, the transducer behavior is dominated mainly by the mass of the moving parts (mass of fluid and that of the piston and spring) and the stiffness (K) of the spring. Recall that if a mass is suspended by a spring, and then the mass is displaced and released, it will oscillate. The frequency of oscillation depends inversely on the mass, and directly on the stiffness. Indeed, this situation applies to the operation of a blood-pressure transducer. However, there is another component that dictates the length of time that the piston (diaphragm) will oscillate when a sudden pressure is applied or removed. This factor is viscous drag that damps the oscillation. Viscous drag results from the friction of the fluid that enters the transducer when pressure is applied. Viscous drag is a force that is proportional to the velocity of fluid movement. Thus, there are three components that conspire to determine the dynamic response of a blood-pressure transducer: 1. mass; 2. stiffness; and 3. viscous drag. The importance of these three components will be examined to show how they dictate the behavior of a blood-pressure transducer to a time-varying hydraulic pressure P(t). The equation of motion that describes the relationship between their three quantities was first solved by Frank (1903, 1912, 1913, 1924).

SINUSOIDAL RESPONSE

It will be shown, subsequently, that the ability of a transducer to respond to a sudden change in pressure is directly related to its natural resonant frequency (f_n) that can be deduced by recalling that for a spring, $f_n = \sqrt{K}/2\pi\sqrt{M}$. For the piston analog of the pressure transducer, $K = A^2/V_d$, where A is the piston area and V_d is the volume displacement (the volume entering the transducer for the application of 100 mm Hg pressure). Substituting for K gives:

$$f_n = \frac{A}{2\pi}\sqrt{\frac{1}{MV_d}}$$

Obviously, it is desirable to design a transducer with a small-dome vol to keep M small, and to have a stiff diaphragm to which provides a small vol displacement (V_d) to achieve a high natural resonant frequency (f_n).

Volume Displacement

The stiffness of a blood pressure transducer diaphragm is described by its volume displacement (V_d), being defined as the number of cubic millimeters of fluid entering the transducer for the application of 100 mm Hg of pressure. Note that this quantity is really a measure of compliance. The smallness of the vol displacement is a figure-of-merit of a transducer. However, because the vol displacement is typically small, it is not accurate to apply 100 mm Hg of fluid pressure and measure the vol of fluid entering the transducer. The reason for not being able to make such an obvious measurement relates to the vol comprehensibility of the fluid filling the transducer dome. A typical dome may contain 1–2 mL of fluid. The compressibility of 1 mL of water at 20°C is 0.006 cubic millimeters for the application of 100 mm Hg. Therefore, if the vol displacement of a transducer is measured by applying 100 mm Hg fluid pressure to the transducer, the vol of fluid entering the transducer is the volume displacement of the transducer plus that caused by the compressibility of the fluid filling the dome. Therefore, another strategy must be used to measure the vol displacement of the transducer alone.

Figure 21 illustrates the method used for the accurate measurement of vol displacement of a blood-pressure transducer. Use of this technique requires only two simple steps

1. The pressure transducer and recording apparatus are calibrated by the application of 100 mm Hg of pressure to the transducer; and
2. The transducer is coupled to a small-bore needle (e.g., 30 ga) and clear plastic tube of small inner diameter (e.g., 0.28 mm).

The transducer dome and plastic tube are filled with colored water, and great care is exercised to exclude all air bubbles. Food coloring dye can be added for easier visualization of the level of the fluid in the clear plastic tube that is viewed with a graticule or lens with a scale placed alongside the plastic tube. Then, an air suction pump is connected to the back (vent) side of the transducer, and a negative pressure of 100 mm Hg is applied. The previously calibrated recording allows identification of the pressure. The colored fluid in the clear plastic tube will fall h units. The vol displacement $= \pi d^2 h/4$, where d is the internal diameter of the clear plastic tube. Of course, more than 100 mm Hg can be used to obtain a better measure of h; but the value of h should be scaled to the one that is produced by 100 mm Hg.

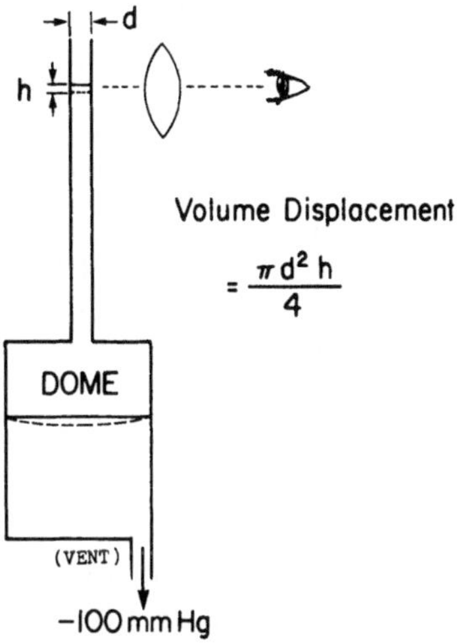

Fig. 21. Method of measuring the volume displacement of a blood-pressure transducent with high accuracy. (Redrawn from Geddes, L. A. et al., *Med. Biol. Eng. Comput.* 1984 (Nov.), 613–614).

Using the method just described, Geddes et al. (1984) measured the volume displacements of several presently used pressure transducers. Table 1 presents the results.

Resonant Frequency

When a sinusoidally varying force is applied to a system with mass, stiffness and damping, the motion that results depends on the frequency of the sine wave and the viscous damping. In the case of a blood-pressure transducer, the resulting motion is the displacement of the diaphragm, and the sinusoidally varying force is represented by hydraulic pressure that is varied sinusoidally. Recall that it was stated earlier, that the behavior of such systems was described by plotting the ratio of the output of the transducer to the input pressure, vs sine wave frequency. The obvious desideratum is to have the ratio of output to input be the same for all frequencies so that the amplitudes of the sinusoidal frequency components in the blood-pressure wave will appear at the transducer output with the same relative amplitudes that they have in the original blood-pressure waveform. In other words, no frequency component should be enhanced or attenuated on passing through the transducer-recording system.

Table 1
Volume Displacement
of Blood Pressure Transducers[a]

Transducer type	Volume displacement (mm^3/100 mm Hg)
Statham P23Db	0.037
Statham P23ID	0.049
Statham P23BB	0.62
Cobe disposable	0.0012

[a]From Geddes, L. A. et al., *Med. Biol. Eng. Comput*. 1984 (Nov.) 613, 614.

When a sinusoidally varying pressure (of frequency f) is applied to a blood pressure transducer, the output depends on the relationship between the frequency f and the natural (undamped) resonant frequency (f_n) and the damping (D). For the spring-loaded piston model (Fig. 16), the natural resonant frequency

$$f_n = \frac{A}{2\pi}\sqrt{\frac{1}{MV_d}}$$

Note that the smaller the mass (M) and the smaller the vol displacement (V_d), the higher the natural resonant frequency. For best reproduction, it is desirable to have a high natural resonant frequency in the transducer.

The damping coefficient (D) is very small in a transducer without a fluid-filled catheter connected to it. Before describing how damping is achieved, it is of value to examine the output of a blood-pressure transducer when different-frequency, constant-amplitude, sinusoidally varying pressure waves are presented to it. Let us assume that the test is made with different degrees of damping. Figure 22 shows the result in which the amplitude of response is plotted vs the ratio of frequency (f) to the natural undamped (resonant) frequency (f_n). It is clear that with very small damping ($D < 0.3$), the amplitude would be extremely large at the natural resonant frequency ($f/f_n = 1.0$). Note also that with $D = 0.707$, the sine-wave frequency response has no rise in it with increasing frequency. Because it is desirable to have the widest sinusoidal frequency response with the minimum rise with increasing frequency, a damping of 0.65 would be preferred.

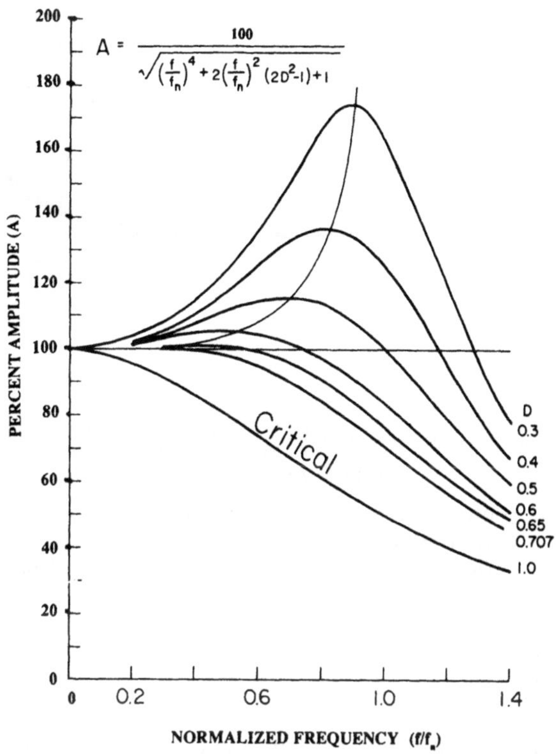

Fig. 22. Percent of amplitude (A) vs frequency for a damped resonant system for various degrees of damping (D). The frequency axis represents the ratio of the frequency (f) used to test the response to the natural resonant frequency (f_n).

Although the foregoing may appear to be only of academic interest, it is not, and provides useful information about blood-pressure transducers. When the hydraulic sine wave frequency response of a transducer only is measured, the result is shown in Fig. 23. Note that the amplitude scale is logarithmic. It is obvious that a transducer by itself is highly underdamped. As we shall see, it is the addition of the fluid-filled catheter that provides the damping, and dramatically alters the performance of the transducer.

Catheter-Transducer Systems

A pressure transducer is coupled to the pressure to be measured by a fluid-filled catheter as shown in Fig. 16B. The addition of this component profoundly alters the performance of the transducer. The use of such a catheter adds two components, mass and viscous

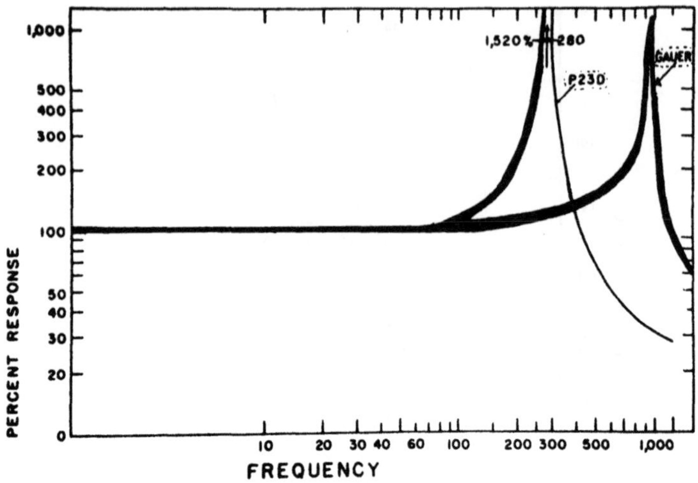

Fig. 23. Output (percent amplitude) vs frequency for one of the popular strain-gauge transducers (Gould-Statham P23) and for a catheter-tip transducer (Gauer and Gienapp, 1950). (Redrawn from Noble, F., URE (IEEE) *Trans. Bio-Med. Eng.* 1957, **PGME 8,** 36–45.)

drag. The latter adds damping because the application of pressure causes fluid to move in the catheter, thereby producing viscous drag. The increased mass of the fluid in the catheter reduces the natural resonant frequency of the system. The way in which the fluid-filled catheter alters the performance characteristics of the transducer will now be discussed.

The mass (M_L) of the fluid in the catheter (Fig. 16B) is equal to its cross sectional area (a) multiplied by its length (L) and the density of (ρ) of the fluid therein; therefore, $M_L = La\rho$. If it is assumed that the flow of fluid in the catheter (owing to the vol displacement of the transducer) is laminar (i.e., nonturbulent), the velocity profile across the catheter diameter is parabolic. This means that fluid particles at the center of the catheter move faster than those near the catheter wall. By summing the kinetic energy of the system, it can be shown that the effective mass of the fluid in the catheter is 4/3 times that of the mass ($M_L = La\rho$) of fluid in the catheter.

The next fact to recognize is that the fluid in the catheter moves A/a times faster than that in the dome of the transducer. Taking these two facts into account, the total effective mass (M_{eq}) of the fluid in the system can be determined by equating kinetic energies as follows

$$\frac{1}{2} M_{eq}\mu^2 = \frac{1}{2}\left(\frac{4M_L}{3}\right)\left(\frac{A}{a}\mu\right)^2 + \frac{1}{2}M\mu^2$$

where μ is the velocity of the fluid in the transducer dome, and the other quantities have been identified previously. Therefore,

$$M_{eq} = \frac{4}{3}\left(\frac{A}{a}\right)^2 M_L + M$$

A differential equation describes the motion of the mass (M_{eq}) that moves with the application of pressure P(t). This equation sums the forces that are 1) mass acceleration, 2) viscous drag and 3) stiffness. The equation is of the form

$$M_{eq}\frac{d^2x}{dt^2} + R\frac{dx}{dt} + \left(\frac{A^2}{V_d}\right)x = P(t)$$

1 MASS ACCELERATION	2 VISCOUS DRAG	3 STIFF-NESS	APPLIED PRESSURE

This equation describes a mass-spring system with viscous damping (Rdx/dt). The importance of the equation lies in the fact that it allows identification of the natural resonant frequency (f_n), that, as stated earlier, allows estimation of the sine-wave frequency response. The natural resonant frequency for a simple mass (M) is

$$f_n = \frac{A}{2\pi}\sqrt{\frac{1}{MV_d}}$$

where A is the area of the diaphragm in the transducer, and V_d is the volume displacement (cu mm/100 mm Hg applied pressure). Therefore, for the effective mass (M_{eq}), the natural resonant frequency is as follows

$$f_n = \frac{A}{2\pi}\sqrt{\frac{1}{V_d\left(M + \frac{4}{3}\left(\frac{A}{a}\right)^2 M_L\right)}}$$

Recall that M is the mass of the fluid in the transducer dome, A and a are the areas of the transducer diaphragm, and the catheter, respectively, and M_L is the mass of the fluid in the catheter that is L cm long. Typically, L is 100 cm, and the diaphragm area (A) is many times larger than the catheter area (a); therefore

$\frac{4}{3}\left(\frac{A}{a}\right)^2 M_L$ is much greater than M. Consequently, the mass of the fluid in the transducer dome can be neglected. The natural resonant frequency now becomes:

$$f_n = \frac{A}{2\pi}\sqrt{\frac{1}{V_d \frac{4}{3}\left(\frac{A}{a}\right)^2 M_L}}$$

Recalling that $a = \pi d^2/4$, where d is the diameter of the catheter,

$$f_n = \frac{d\sqrt{3}}{8\sqrt{\pi \rho L \, V_d}}$$

From the foregoing, it can be seen that the mass of the fluid in the catheter dominates that of the fluid in the transducer dome. Moreover, the natural resonant frequency (f_n) decreases with increasing catheter length (L). Note that the internal diameter (d) and length (L) of the catheter are dictated by the particular measurement conditions. Therefore, the only way to achieve a high natural resonant frequency is to choose a transducer with a small vol displacement (V_d). Recall that it is the natural resonant frequency (along with damping), that defines the sine-wave frequency response (Fig. 22).

Damping

Although the attainment of a high natural resonant frequency is a primary desideratum, provision of the desired degree of damping is another. Therefore, it is important to identify those factors that control the viscous drag or damping. The damping coefficient (D) can be found by solving the differential equation that governs the motion of the transducer diaphragm and applying Poiseuille's law, that relates pressure, flow, fluid viscosity (n), length (L), and diameter (d) of the catheter. For a system of which the effective mass of the fluid in the catheter is greater than that in the transducer dome, the damping coefficient (D) is given by

$$D = \frac{16n}{d^3}\sqrt{\frac{3LV_d}{\pi \rho}}$$

where L and d are catheter length and diameter, ρ and n are the density and viscosity of the fluid in the catheter, and V_d is the transducer vol displacement.

It is important to recognize that the foregoing was derived assuming that the catheter was stiff-walled, i.e., the vol displacement of the catheter was zero. If the catheter is made of compliant material, the application of pressure will distend its wall and the volume displacement will be large, resulting in increased damping.

Converting the damping expression to permit its use with practical units of measurement in which the catheter length (L) is in cm., its diameter (d) is in mm, the vol displacement V_d is in cu mm/100 mm Hg, and water has a density of 1.0 gm/mL and a viscosity of 0.01 poise, yields

$$D = \frac{0.135\sqrt{LV_d}}{d^3}$$

Again it is well to remember that the foregoing equation was developed using the spring-loaded piston analog (Fig. 16), and assumes that an ideal, stiff-walled catheter was used. Real catheters (Table 2) do not have a rigid wall, thereby increasing the vol displacement. Consequently, the measured damping will be slightly higher than that predicted by the foregoing equation.

The practical consequence of adding a fluid-filled catheter to a transducer is shown in Fig. 24. It can be seen that the addition of the catheter reduced the resonant frequency and increased the damping, as evidenced by the reduced amplitude for the damped resonant frequency. Compare this response to that predicted in Fig. 22.

An excellent way of demonstrating the effect of increasing damping without changing the mass of a system is shown in Fig. 25. To make this illustration, blood pressure was recorded with a transducer connected to a fluid filled catheter in the femoral artery of a dog. Then, the diameter of the catheter was decreased by gradually squeezing it between the jaws of a hemostat. The small fluid flow into and out of the transducer encounters an ever increasing resistance at the point where the catheter is pinched, thereby increasing the viscous drag and damping. Note that the dicrotic notch disappears first, and then the pulse amplitude decreases and virtually disappears, the record then displaying mean pressure.

The procedure just described is easy to perform, and is illuminating for several reasons. For example, as shown in Fig. 22, increasing damping decreases the sine wave frequency response.

Table 2
Catheter Dimensions*

Material and French size[1]	Lumen mm	Lumen in	Outside diameter mm	Outside diameter in	Color
Teflon					
T3.0	0.58	.023	1.00	.040	Gray
T4.0	0.74	.029	1.33	.052	Gray
T5.0	0.99	.039	1.66	.066	Gray
T6.3	1.37	.054	2.10	.083	Gray
TW6.4	1.60	.063	2.13	.084	White
T6.5	1.45	.057	2.16	.085	Gray
T7.0	1.57	.062	2.33	.092	Gray
T8.0	1.83	.072	2.66	.105	Gray
T9.0	2.08	.082	3.00	.118	Gray
Polyethylene					
P3.0	0.56	.022	1.00	.040	Green
P3.7	0.74	.029	1.23	.048	Yellow
P4.0	0.69	.027	1.33	.052	Red
P4.1	0.94	.037	1.36	.054	Green
P5.0	1.06	.042	1.66	.066	Red
P5.0B[2]	1.12	.044	1.66	.066	White
P5.0M[3]	1.12	.044	1.66	.066	Gray
P5.2	1.09	.043	1.73	.068	Green
P5.3C	1.17	.046	1.76	.069	Yellow
P6.0	1.19	.047	2.00	.079	Black
P6.3	1.50	.059	2.10	.083	Green
P6.5	1.47	.058	2.16	.085	Red
P6.7	1.50	.059	2.23	.088	Yellow
P7.0	1.27	.050	2.33	.092	Black
P7.1	1.57	.062	2.36	.093	Red
P7.2	1.47	.058	2.40	.094	Green
P8.0	1.55	.061	2.66	.105	Black
P8.0S[4]	1.75	.069	2.66	.105	Green
P8.3	1.52	.060	2.76	.109	Yellow
P8.3G[4]	1.78	.070	2.76	.109	Gray
P9.0	1.83	.072	3.00	.118	Black

Note, the number following the letter is the French (F) size. The outer diameter in mm is the F size divided by three.

*Courtesy, Cook Inc., Bloomington, IN.

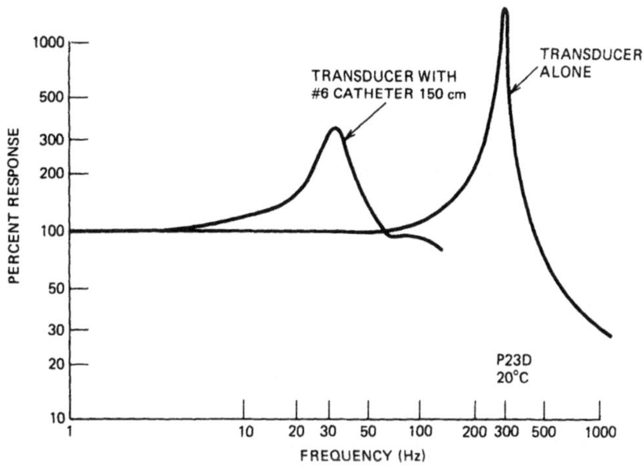

Fig. 24. Sine wave frequency response of a P23D (Statham) transducer, and the sine wave frequency response for the same transducer connected to a 6F catheter, 150 cm long. Note that addition of the fluid-filled catheter increased the damping, and reduced the frequency of the resonant peak in the sine wave frequency response. (Redrawn from Noble, F. IRE (IEEE) *Trans. Bio-Med. Eng.* 1957, **PGME 8,** 36–45.)

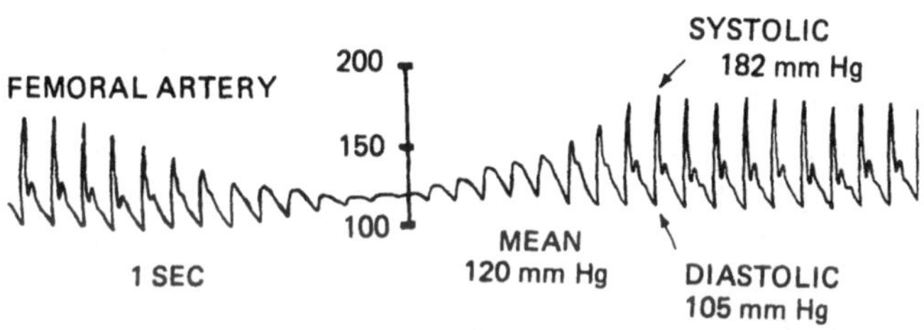

Fig. 25. Mean pressure obtained by diminishing the ability of the recording system to follow rapid changes. Mean pressure was revealed by gradually clamping the catheter leading to a high-fidelity pressure transducer. (From Geddes, L. A., *Cardiovascular Devices,* New York, 1984, John Wiley. By permission.)

Since the dicrotic notch contains the highest frequency components, decreasing the sine wave response makes the notch less sharp, and a further reduction in high frequency response makes it disappear. With increased damping, the frequency response becomes so poor that not even the fundamental (the sine wave that corresponds to the cardiac frequency) can no longer be reproduced, and the pulse pressure becomes smaller and smaller with increasing damping. Finally, the sine wave frequency response becomes so poor that only the mean pressure can be reproduced.

TRANSIENT RESPONSE

The foregoing has dealt with steady-state conditions in which each cycle is the same as the next. However, the foregoing concepts are easily generalized to accommodate the response to a transient, i.e., a sudden change that is not periodic. A transient can be described as a sudden change from one value to another. Such a waveform is called a step function. Figure 26 illustrates this type of signal that is easy to generate electronically. Figure 26A illustrates a positive step function, and Fig. 26B illustrates a negative step function. It should be obvious that the nature of the dynamic response of a system can be revealed with either waveform. To date, creating a positive pressure transient to test the dynamic response of a catheter-transducer system has been difficult. Nonetheless, a simple method has been found to generate a negative pressure transient. Prior to describing this method of testing, a catheter-transducer system, the way in which the natural resonant frequency and damping determine the ability to respond to a step-function change in pressure must be presented. By putting P(t) equal to the step function (Fig. 26B), and solving the differential equation, it is possible to determine the response of a catheter-transducer system to the sudden removal of a sustained pressure.

It can be anticipated that if a steady pressure is removed from the catheter tip, the elastic recoil of the deflected transducer diaphragm will cause a small amount of fluid to move out of the catheter tip. Therefore, a mass is driven by a force, and viscous drag impairs recoil of the transducer diaphragm. Figure 27 illustrates the response of a system in which the damping (D) is 0.2, 0.5, 0.7, and 1.0 (critical damping). Two observations need to be made. 1. The less the damping, the larger the undershoot and; and 2. The less the damping, the more rapid the return to the position of equilibrium. In other words, increasing damping decreases the undershoot and oscillations (ringing) and prolongs the response time, i.e., the time taken to return to the equilibrium level. Note that with critical damping (D = 1.0), there is no undershoot, but the time to return to the equilibrium level is very long.

At this point, it is appropriate to recall how the sinusoidal frequency response (Fig. 22) is affected by damping. For the faithful reproduction of a waveform, all of the sinusoidal frequency components must be reproduced with the same relative amplitudes as they existed in the complex wave. This means that a uniform (flat) sinusoidal frequency response is required. From Fig. 27, it is seen that

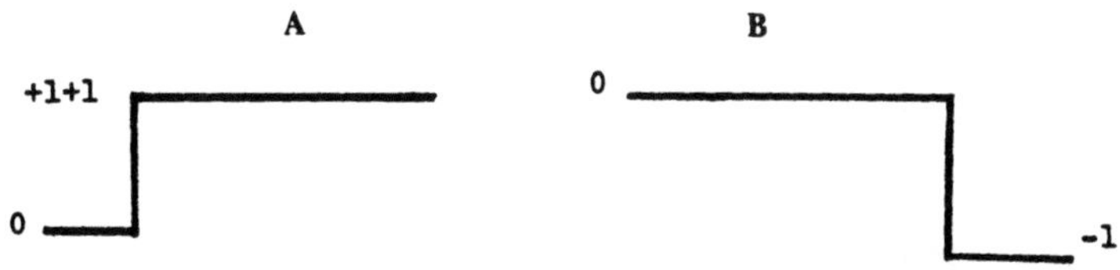

Fig. 26. The step function; A illustrates a positive-going step function of amplitude +1, and B illustrates the sudden removal of a preexisting signal of amplitude +1.

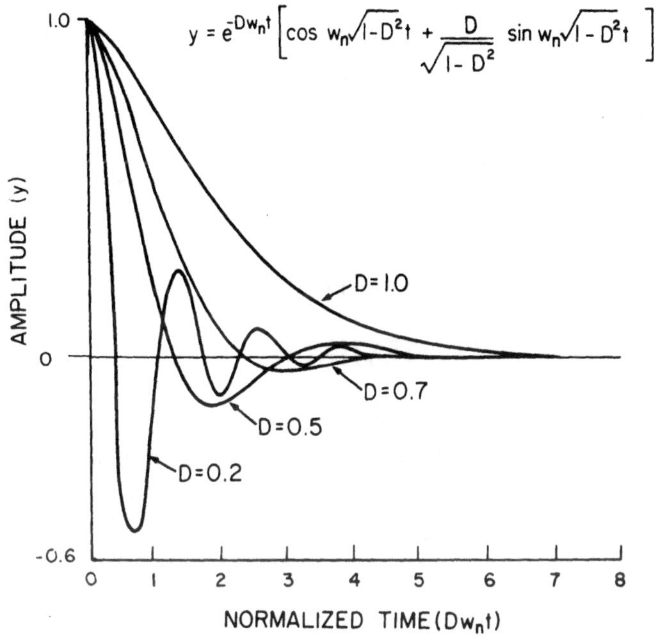

Fig. 27. Response of a catheter-transducer system by suddenly removing a constant pressure (1.0). ($\omega_n = 2\pi f_n t$)

a damping factor of about 0.7 provided this requirement. Referring to Fig. 28, it is seen that a 4.6% undershoot in response to a step function is obtained with this damping. Therefore, a catheter-transducer system should be designed to achieve this degree of damping. Whether this is attained in practice can be determined by the test that will soon be described.

Figure 28 shows the percent undershoot (or overshoot) that will be obtained when a step function of pressure is removed (or applied) to a catheter-transducer system with different degrees of damping. In viewing this relationship, it should be recalled that increasing the damping (D) prolongs the rise time.

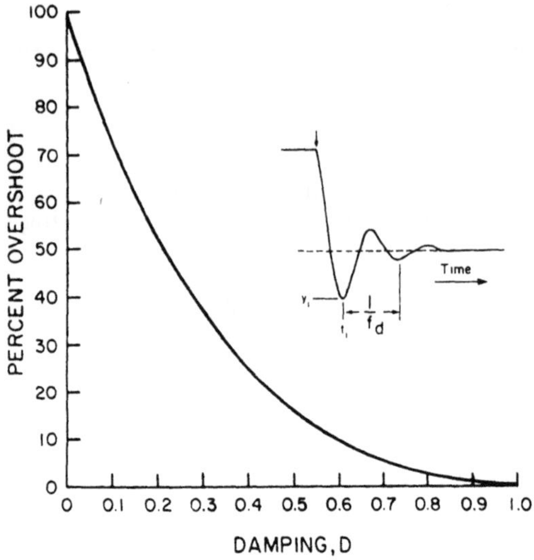

Fig. 28. Percent undershoot vs damping (D).

DYNAMIC RESPONSE TESTING

Geddes and Bourland (1988) described an easily applied method for testing the dynamic response of a catheter-transducer system. The method is illustrated in Fig. 29. It is imperative that the transducer and catheter be filled with fluid, and that no air bubbles are present in the entire system. Often, the addition of a little alcohol to the fluid facilitates filling without air bubbles. Even the tiniest air bubble increases the vol displacement and increases the damping.

The test is easily performed when the entire system is fluid filled by first turning the three-way stopcock so that the water bottle is in communication with the transducer. Then, the bottle is pressurized to 100 mm Hg and the stopcock is closed, trapping the 100 mm Hg in the catheter and transducer. The recording system is turned to its maximum speed and the stopcock is opened suddenly to allow the catheter to communicate with atmospheric pressure. This maneuver causes the pressure to fall from 100 mm Hg to zero, and the dynamic response of the catheter-transducer system will be revealed by the graphic recorder. It is important to use a graphic recorder with a rapid response time, i.e., one that is shorter than 10 ms, that is equivalent to a sine wave frequency response better than 0–50 Hz. If it is suspected that the electronic recorder may not have an adequately short response time, the step-function test can be applied by presenting a voltage to its input terminals. For example,

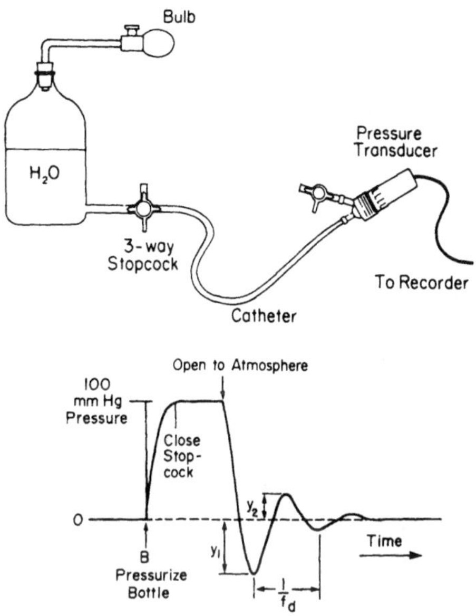

Fig. 29. Method used to test the dynamic response of a fluid-filled, catheter-transducer system. The test consists of applying 100 mm Hg to the fluid in the water-filled bottle in communication with the catheter. Then, the 3-way stopcock is closed, entrapping the pressure in the catheter. The response is obtained by suddenly opening the stopcock to atmospheric pressure.

the transducer is disconnected and a 50 μV signal is suddenly applied. This voltage represents about 60 mm Hg for a typical transducer. Such a signal can be obtained by connecting a voltage divider of 1/30,000 across a 1.5 volt battery when observing the recorded display, and measuring the time for 0 to 100% response.

Figure 30 is an example of a dynamic response test with a water-filled 7F catheter, 100 cm long, connected to a Statham P23db pressure transducer. Note that the response time (0–100%) is 25 ms, and the undershoot is 11.5%. The damped resonant frequency (f_d) is 20 Hz. This undershoot indicates that the damping D = 0.57 (Fig. 27).

The dynamic test just described is often called the pop test. It can be used with catheters of any size and length connected to any of the presently used pressure transducers. It is essential to open the stopcock quickly so that a sudden drop in pressure is presented to the catheter-transducer system.

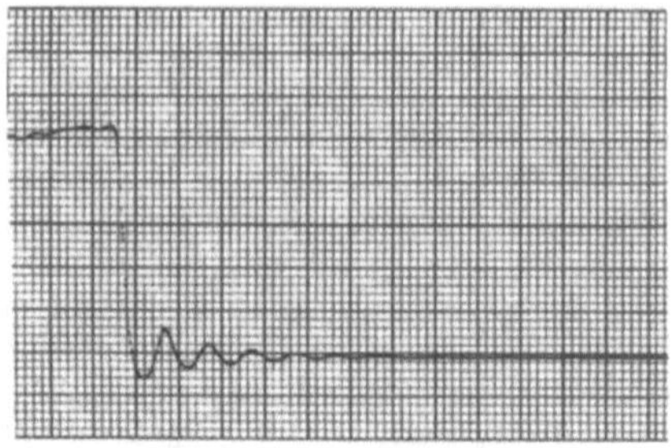

Fig. 30. Response of a blood pressure transducer (Gould-Statham P23db) connected to a #7F fluid-filled catheter, one meter long. (Time scale 1 div. = 0.01 s) (From Geddes, L. A. and Bourland, J. D., *Journ. Clin. Eng.* 1988, Jan–Feb 59–62) (by permission).

Catheter Whip

Even with a catheter and transducer matched to provide a uniform sinusoidal frequency response, it is possible to record blood pressure waves that are distorted if the catheter flails in the vessel or chamber wherein pressure is measured. Such flailing produces accelerative forces in the fluid in the catheter, the result being spurious pressure changes. Catheter whip is the term often used to describe this type of artifact.

Noble (1957) published a record of catheter whip, encountered with the tip of a 6F catheter, 150 cm long, in the pulmonary artery of a dog. The catheter was connected to a Statham P23D pressure transducer. To show that the pressure recording contained catheter whip artifacts, he recorded pressure at the same site with a Gauer (1950) catheter-tip transducer, demonstrating clearly that the pressure in the pulmonary artery did not contain the oscillations detected by the fluid-filled catheter transducer system (Fig. 31).

Another example of catheter whip is shown in Fig. 31E. To make this illustration, Piemme (1963) coupled a 5F Teflon catheter to a strain gauge transducer. The tip of the catheter was located in a region of high flow velocity to produce the catheter-whip artifact shown in Fig. 31E. The true pressure waveform (Fig. 31D) was obtained with a second strain gauge transducer and catheter, the tip of which was not in a region of high flow velocity. In Fig. 31C is shown the ECG for reference purposes.

The foregoing clearly demonstrates that spurious waveforms can be generated with a properly designed and correctly operating pressure-recording system.

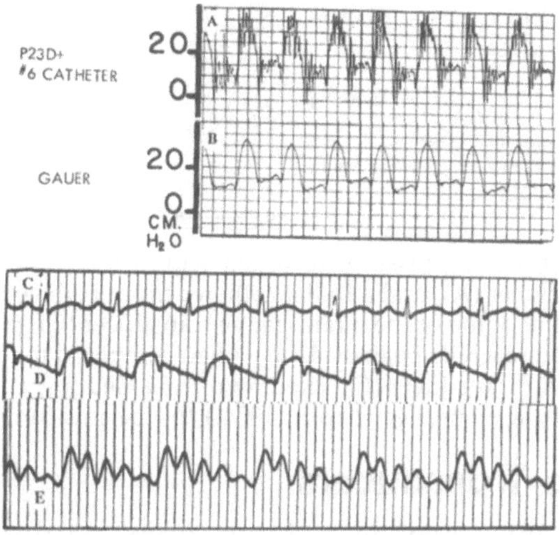

Fig. 31. Examples of distortion caused by catheter whip. In A is shown a record of pulmonary artery pressure in the dog, made with a 6F catheter, 150 cm long, connected to a P23D Statham pressure transducer. In B is shown pressure at the same site, recorded with a catheter-tip (Gauer) pressure transducer. In C is shown the ECG and blood pressure (D), recorded with the catheter tip not in a high flow velocity, and with a second catheter with its tip in a high flow velocity region (E). (A and B redrawn from Noble, F., IEEE *Trans. Biomed Eng.* 1957, **PGME8,** 38–45. C, D, and E are redrawn from Piemme, T. E., *Prog. Cardiovasc. Dev.* 1963, **5,** 574–594.)

Air Bubbles

Air is compressible, and the presence of even a tiny air bubble increases the vol displacement of a catheter-transducer system, leading to increased damping and a prolonged response time. The consequence of adding a very small air bubble to the fluid in the dome of a pressure transducer is shown in Fig. 32. On the left is shown the carotid artery pressure recorded with a strain-gauge transducer connected to a 6F catheter (A) and a Millar catheter-tip pressure transducer (B). On the right (C) is shown the recording made with a tiny air bubble injected into the dome of the transducer; below (D) is shown a simultaneously obtained record with the catheter-tip transducer. Note that although the waveforms in C and D are very similar, addition of the air bubble increased the damping, and prolonged the time for the waveform to reach its peak by 42 ms.

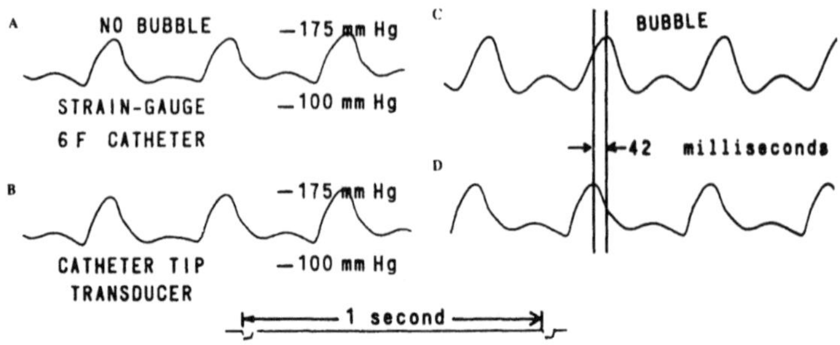

Fig. 32. Carotid artery pressure, recorded with a 6 F catheter connected to a strain-gauge transducer (A), and a Millar catheter-tip transducer (B). A tiny bubble was injected into the dome of the strain-gauge transducer (C), prolonging the time for the waveform to reach its peak by 42 ms when compared to the record obtained with the catheter-tip transducer (D). (Redrawn from Geddes, L. A., *Cardiovascular Devices,* John Wiley & Sons, New York, 1984.) (by permission)

Catheter-Tip Transducers

Several important advantages derive from locating the pressure transducer at the tip of the catheter. For example, the long fluid column with its considerable effective mass and viscous drag are eliminated. The transducer diaphragm at the catheter tip is very small, lightweight, and stiff. All of these factors conspire to provide a high natural resonant frequency and low damping. Resonant frequencies of 1000 Hz are not uncommon (Fig. 23). The result of these factors is to provide a very rapid response time and the ability to reproduce rapidly changing pressures.

The idea of locating the transducer at the catheter tip is not new. Grunbaum (1897, 1898) constructed an electrolytic transducer located on the side at the tip of a 3 mm diameter catheter. With it, he recorded right-ventricular pressure in the rabbit.

Despite Grunbaum's success, catheter-tip pressure transducers were not to reappear until the 1940s when Wetterer (1943) described a variable inductance unit with a tip diameter of 3.5 mm. A differential-transformer transducer with a 2.7 mm tip diameter was developed by Gauer and Gienapp (1950). This unit was rugged and enjoyed considerable success in aeromedical research. In 1962, Allard developed a variable inductance, catheter-tip pressure transducer with a proximal sampling port. This device was available for a short time. (Carolina Medical Electronics, Winston-Salem, NC). At about the same time, Statham Medical Instruments (Oxnard, CA) introduced a strain-gauge, catheter-tip pressure transducer with an angled tip. Although it worked well, it had a short lifetime.

These early catheter-tip transducers all performed satisfactorily, but they were not embraced with much enthusiasm, probably for two reasons. Each required special equipment for operation, and the signal produced was quite small. Soon, strain-gauge elements became available having a large resistance change with extension. The first catheter-tip (7F) transducer using such elements was described by Angelakos (1964). However, the turning point in the acceptance of catheter-tip transducers came in 1969 when Huntly Millar started development of a rugged, easy-to-use, catheter tip, strain-gauge pressure transducer in his home laboratory in Houston, TX. One of these units is shown in Fig. 33; it has remarkably good performance characteristics, namely, a high output per mm Hg, and an extremely short response time (i.e., excellent high-frequency response). Millar and Baker (1973) presented the first paper describing the Millar MIKRO-TIP catheter-tip pressure transducer that has become the standard in the field today. Millar has also developed a disposable, catheter-tip, strain-gauge pressure transducer. Others are developing disposable units of various designs.

Figure 33 illustrates a record of right-ventricular pressure and its rate of change (dP/dt). Note that the Millar transducer is side-viewing for pressure measurement.

It was stated earlier that catheter-tip pressure transducers have a wide frequency response owing to their high natural frequency. To illustrate this point, Fig. 34 is presented that displays aortic pressure, left ventricular pressure, and the ECG of a patient with severe aortic stenosis. Note the large difference between the left ventricular and aortic pressures. The stenotic sound (aortic phono) recording was made by amplifying the output of the transducer on the catheter that was used to display aortic pressure. In other words, this pressure transducer served as a microphone.

Catheter-tip pressure transducers provide an accurate reproduction of hemodynamic waveforms. However, until the advent of multi-sensor catheters, it had not been possible to obtain high-fidelity comparisons of pressures at different locations in the heart or vascular system. In 1972, Millar developed the first dual pressure sensor catheter, with sensors 5 cm apart, for measurement of pressures across the aortic valve in man (Fig. 34). This catheter permitted calculation of instantaneous flow through the aortic valve by the pressure-gradient technique. Obviously, such a unit can be used to measure the pressure drop across a stenosis in a blood vessel.

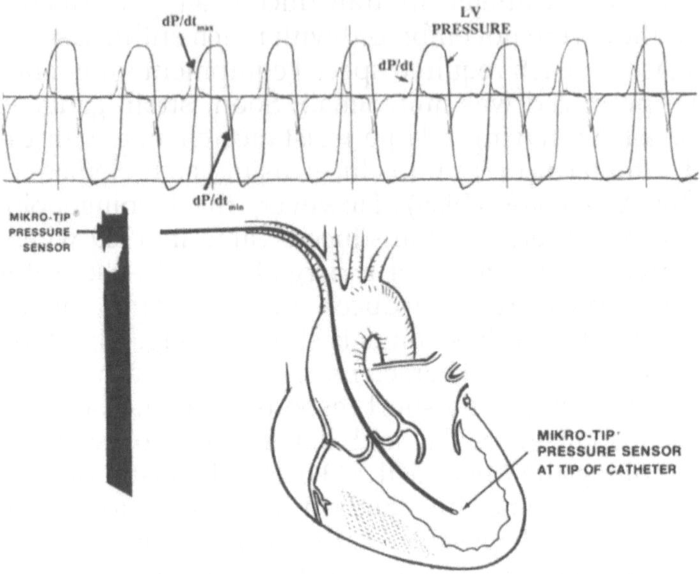

Fig. 33. The Millar Mikro-Tip pressure transducer. (Courtesy, Millar Instruments, Houston, TX.)

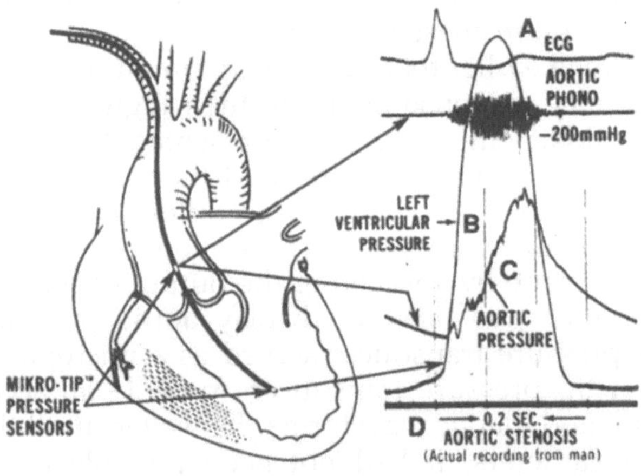

Fig. 34. The ECG (A), left ventricular pressure (B), aortic pressure (C), and the sounds of aortic stenoses (D). The latter made by amplifying and high-pass filtering the output of the pressure transducer used to measure aortic pressure (Courtesy, Millar Instruments, Houston, TX.)

In January, 1973, Millar cooperated with Carolina Medical Electronics to produce a catheter combining the Millar pressure sensor with the Carolina electromagnetic catheter velocity probe. Subsequently, Millar developed an electromagnetic velocity probe with a pressure sensor at the same location, permitting simultaneous correlation of pressure and flow at one point in the circulatory system. Further development led to a catheter specifically for the right side of the heart for simultaneously measuring pressure and flow velocity in the pulmonary artery, as well as pressures in the right ventricle and right atrium. Another catheter, designed for the left side of the heart, measured left-ventricular pressure and velocity in the aorta.

Multisensor catheters are presently available in many configurations (Fig. 35) for use in cardiology, urology, gastroenterology, and esophageal manometry.

Further miniaturization extended these high fidelity studies to the coronary arteries. In 1986, Millar introduced a miniature (3F), 20-MHz Doppler-tipped catheter transducer for measuring blood flow velocity and pressure in the coronary arteries. Recent technology has permitted the construction of a 2F catheter with a single MIKRO-TIP pressure sensor and a size 3F catheter with two pressure sensors for measuring pressures across a coronary artery stenosis.

Rate of Change of Pressure (dP/dt)

The rate of change of pressure (dP/dt) is the slope of the pressure-time waveform at a given point; the units are mm Hg/s. Figure 33 illustrates left ventricular pressure and its rate of change (dP/dt). Note that just after the onset of ventricular contraction, dP/dt reaches its maximum (dP/dt_{max}) and then decreases. Just after the onset of relaxation, the rate of change of pressure reaches its minimum (dP/dt_{min}). A continuous record of dP/dt is obtained by electronic differentiation of the pressure waveform. Although it would be desirable to record left ventricular dP/dt continuously, this is often impractical and dP/dt of the arterial pressure waveform is often used instead.

The maximum rate of increase in pressure (dP/dt_{max}) reflects the vigor of ventricular contraction. For this reason, there was considerable interest in this quantity, and it was thought that there was a normal range, and that values beyond this range would be

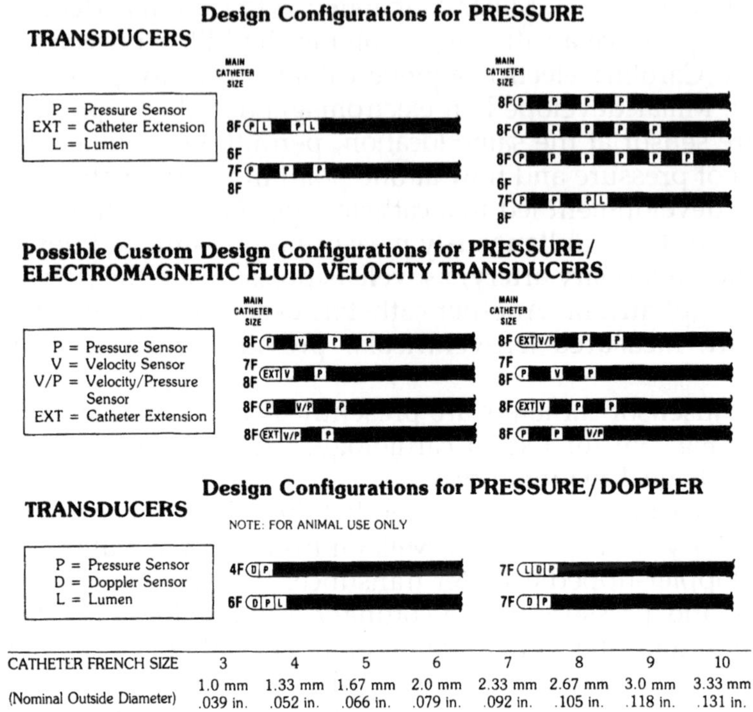

Fig. 35. Various catheter-tip pressure transducers and flowmeters presently available (Courtesy, Millar Instruments, Houston, TX).

used as diagnostic information. It timed out that there is a considerable range for dP/dt_{max}. However, if during a recording session this quantity starts to decrease, it is cause for seeking the reason for the decrease in contractility.

Calibration of the dP/dt Record

There are two methods for calibrating the dP/dt channel. Because it is impractical to generate an hydraulic pressure change at a selected rate, recourse is taken to the use of an electrical method. Either a triangular or a sine wave can be used to provide the calibrating signal.

Triangular-Wave Calibration

The first step in calibrating a dP/dt channel consists of adjusting the recording system to obtain a pressure recording and a dP/dt recording of satisfactory amplitude as shown in Fig. 36A and B, respectively. Then, without altering any controls in the recording channels, known pressures are applied to callibrate the pressure recording as shown in Fig. 36A. Then, the pressure transducer is disconnected, and a low-frequency (e.g., 2 Hz) triangular-wave signal is fed into the pressure-recording channel as shown in Fig. 36C. The amplitude of this new input signal is increased so that suitably large amplitude recording is obtained, e.g., a peak-to-peak amplitude equivalent to 100 mm Hg, as shown in Fig. 36D. Note that the dP/dt channel produces a square wave (Fig. 36D) because the slope of a triangular wave is constant. In Fig. 36C, the peak-to-peak pressure is 100 mm Hg, and the frequency of the triangular wave is 2 Hz. This means that the rate of pressure rise is 100 mm Hg in 0.25 s or + 400 mm Hg s. Similarly, the rate of pressure fall is −100 mm Hg/0.25 s = −400 mm Hg/s. Thus, the dP/dt channel rises to +400, and falls to −400 mm Hg/s as shown in Fig. 36D, and the zero level for dP/dt is midway between these two values. It is noteworthy that this recorded triangular wave signal, although not derived from a pressure source, can be used to simulate a changing pressure signal.

Sine Wave Calibration

Sine-wave generators are usually more common than triangular-wave generators, and the sine-wave calibration method will now be described. The first step is to adjust the recorder for satisfactory recordings as shown in Fig. 37 A and B. Then, the pressure channel is calibrated with known pressures as shown in Fig. 37A. Without altering any controls, the pressure transducer is disconnected, and a low frequency (e.g., 4 Hz) sine-wave generator is connected to the pressure-recording channel. The peak-to-peak output of the sine wave generator is adjusted to obtain a satisfactorily large amplitude pressure wave, e.g., 100 mm Hg, as shown in Fig. 37C. When this is done, the dP/dt channel records a cosine wave (Fig. 37D), and the peak-to-peak amplitude allows calibration of the dP/dt channel.

Consider a sine wave of pressure having a frequency f and a peak value P_m; mathematically, this wave is expressed as $P_m \sin 2\pi ft$, where t is time. The derivative of $P_m \sin 2\pi ft$ is as follows

$$\frac{d}{dt}(P_m \sin 2\pi ft) = 2\pi f P_m (\cos 2\pi ft)$$

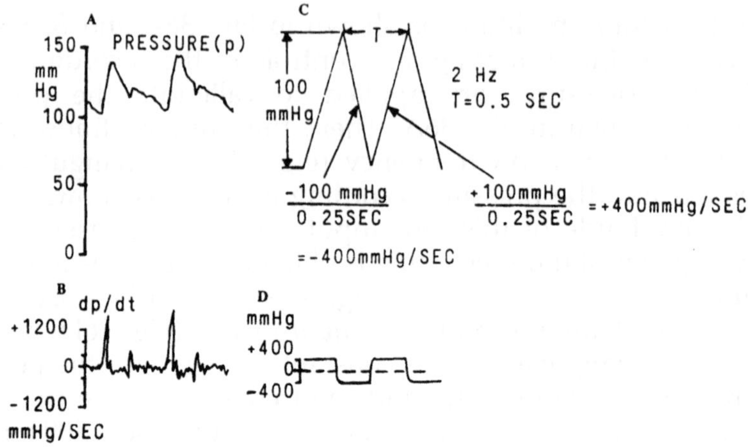

Fig. 36. Arterial pressure (A) and its derivative (B), and the triangular wave methods (D), used for calibration.

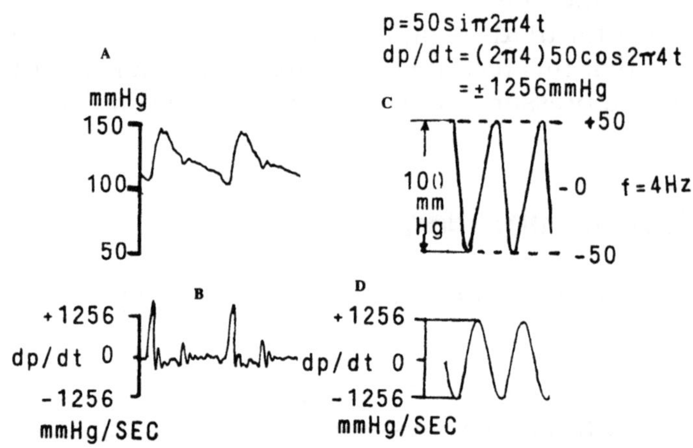

Fig. 37. Arterial pressure (A), its derivative (B), and the sine wave method (C,D), used for calibration.

Therefore, the peak amplitude of the derivative (dP/dt) channel is $2\pi f$ times the peak amplitude of the pressure channel (=50 mm Hg).

The calibrating 4-Hz sine wave amplitude was adjusted to 100 mm Hg peak-to-peak. This means that the pressure channel oscillated between ± 50 mm Hg. The positive amplitude of the derivative channel is $50(2\pi\ 4) = 400\ \pi$ or 1256 mm Hg/s. Similarly, the dP/dt channel has a negative amplitude of 1256 mm Hg as shown in Fig. 37D. These calibration amplitudes are applied to the dP/dt channel as shown in Fig. 37B.

REFERENCES

Allard, E. M. Sound and pressure signals obtained from a single intracardiac catheter, IRE Trans. on Biomed. Electronics *BME* 1962, **9,** 74–77,

Angelakos, E. T. Semiconductor pressure transducers. *Amer. Journ. Med. Elect.* 1964–65, **34,** 266–270.

Frank, O. Kritik der elastichen Manometer. *Zeits. f. Biol.* 1903, **44,** 445–613; 1912, 1913, **59,** 526–530; and 1924, **82,** 49–65.

Gauer, O. H. and Gienapp, E. A. Miniature pressure recording device. *Science* 1950, **112,** 404–405.

Geddes, L. A. Technical Note: The Significance of a reference in the direct measurement of blood pressure. *Journ. Med. Instr.* 1986, **20(6),** 331, 332. Also, *Journ. Clin. Eng.* 1986, **11,** 481, 482 (Publisher's error).

Geddes, L. A., Athens, W., and Aronson, S. Measurement of the volume displacement of blood pressure transducers. *Med. Biol. Eng. Comput.* 1984, (Nov), 613, 614.

Geddes, L. A. and Bourland, J. D. Estimation of the damping coefficient of fluid-filled, catheter transducer, /pressure-measuring systems. *Journ. Clin. Eng.* 1988, Jan–Feb. 59–62.

Grunbaum, O. F. On a new method of recording alterations of pressure. *Journ. Physiol.* 1897–1898, **22,** XLiX–Li.

Hales, S. Statical Essays. *Haemostaticks,* vol. 2 (3rd Ed.), London, 1738. W. Innys and R. Manby. 341 pp.

Lambert, E. H. and Wood, E. H. The use of a resistance wire strain gauge manometer to measure intraarterial pressure. *Proc. Soc. Exp. Biol. Med.* 1947, **64,** 186–190.

Millar, H. D. and Baker, L. E. A stable ultraminiature catheter tip transducer. *Med. Biol. Eng. Comput.* 1973, **11(1),** 86–89.

Noble, F. The sonic valve pressure transducer. IRE (IEEE) *Trans. Bio-Med. Eng.* 1957, **PGME 8,** 36–45.

Piemme, T. E. Pressure measurement: electrical pressure transducers. *Prog. Cardiovasc. Dis.* 1963, **5,** 574–594.

Poiseuille, J. L. M. Rescherches sur la force du coeur aortique. *Archiv. Gen. de Med.* 1828, **18,** 550–555.

Poiseuille, J. L. M. *La Force du Coeur Aortique.* Thesis presented to the Faculty of Medicine, Univ. Paris, Aug. 8. 1828. Paris, 1828 Didiot le Jeune.

Voelz, M. Measurement of the blood-pressure constant K. *Med. Biol. Eng. Comput.* 1981, **19,** 535–537.

Wetterer, E. Eine neue manometrische Sonde mit elektrischer Transmission, *Zschr. Biol.* 1943, **101,** 332–350.

PART TWO

The Indirect Measurement of Blood Pressure

INTRODUCTION

One hundred twenty over eighty (120/80) and 90 mm Hg diastolic pressure are the numbers of interest to the general public and the cardiologist, respectively. The former (120/80) is a comfortable target for most people; 90 mm Hg diastolic is the flag for seeking signs of hypertension. As is well known, blood pressure increases with age in males and females; Fig. 1 illustrates this point.

Whether the measured pressure is 120/80, or the diastolic pressure is 90 mm Hg depends on the method used to make the measurement, as well as the operator's technique and the particular instant in the respiratory cycle when the measurement is made (in the absence of an arrhythmia). Even at rest, blood pressure is not constant. Respiration modulates it from a few to about 10 mm Hg or more, if the breathing is slow and deep. In a study of 25 patients, Hochberg (1971) quantitated the respiratory variation in nonarrhythmic subjects and found that 50% or more of the subjects exhibited a 10.5 mm Hg variation in systolic, and a 12 mm Hg variation in diastolic pressure.

A component of the respiratory variation in blood pressure is owing to the normal variation in heart rate with respiration. Moreover, vasomotor (Traube-Hering) waves, usually occurring with a frequency of 4 to 7 per min, can often be encountered in hypoxia. If an arrhythmia is present, the variation in blood pressure can be considerable, making it difficult to obtain consistent values.

There are many methods of measuring blood pressure noninvasively. All employ an inflatable cuff to apply a counterpressure to

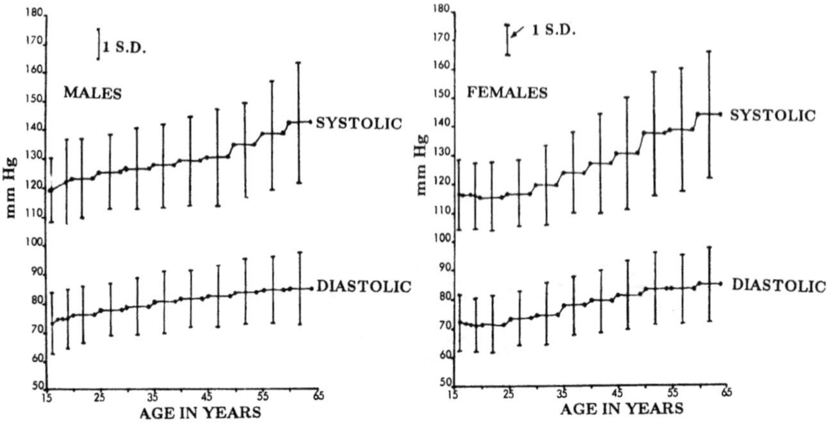

Fig. 1. Normal values for blood pressure in the human, according to age and sex. (Plotted from data in Master, A. M. et al.; *Normal Blood Pressure and Hypertension*, Lea & Febiger, Philadelphia, 1952, with permission.)

occlude an underlying artery that is slowly relieved of the counterpressure by gradual cuff deflation. The various methods are listed in Table 1, along with the pressures that they measure. The palpatory and the flush methods employ an indicator of return of the pulse during cuff deflation from above systolic pressure. The auscultatory method employs the appearance and disappearance of Korotkoff sounds during cuff deflation. The oscillometric method employs the amplitude of cuff-pressure oscillations to indicate systolic, mean, and diastolic pressures. The ultrasonic method uses detection of the vessel-wall movements during cuff deflation.

Many studies have been conducted with a view to using the velocity of the arterial pulse wave to determine blood pressure. Pulse-wave velocity depends on blood pressure, and tracks its change quite well. However, to date, it has not been possible to calibrate pulse-wave velocity in terms of mm Hg; although a considerable research effort in this direction is underway.

THE CUFF

All clinically used indirect methods of measuring blood pressure employ time sampling, and do not permit continuous measurement. In other words, the blood pressure cuff is deflated at a constant rate or incrementally, as shown in Fig. 2. The ability to identify systolic, mean, and diastolic pressures accurately depends on the method employed and the rate of cuff deflation relative to heart rate. With a constant heart rate and a linear decrease in cuff

Table 1
Indirect Methods of Measuring Blood Pressure

Method	Systolic	Mean	Diastolic
Palpatory	Yes	No	No
Flush	Yes	No	No
Auscultatory	Yes	Yes[a]	Yes
Oscillometric	Yes[b]	Yes	Yes[b]
Ultrasonic	Yes	No	Yes

[a]Under investigation
[b]Derived values

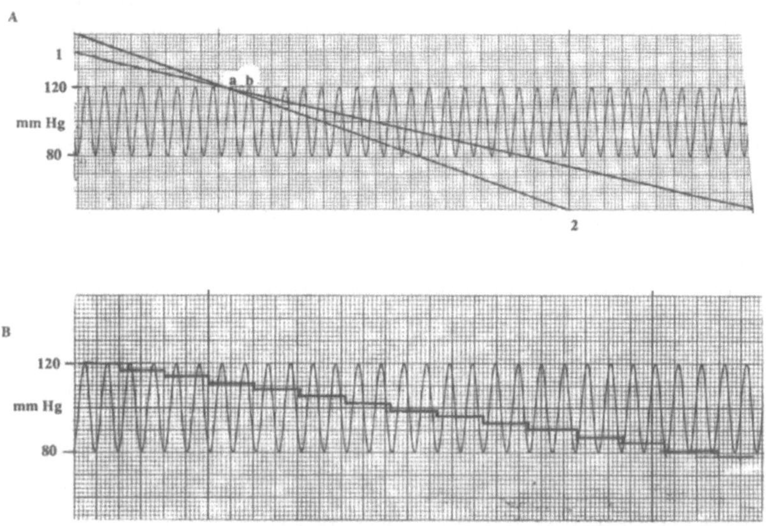

Fig. 2. The constant-rate method of cuff deflation (A), and the incremental method (B).

pressure (using, for example, the auscultatory method to identify systolic and diastolic pressures), the instant when cuff pressure falls below systolic and diastolic pressures, depends on cuff deflation rate. For example, for pulse a in Fig. 2A, cuff pressure intersects systolic pressure, and no Korotkoff sound would be heard. For pulse b, cuff pressure intersected the arterial pulse just below systolic pressure, and a sound would be heard. The American Heart Association (AHA) (1980) recommends a cuff-deflation rate of 3mm Hg/s. For a heart rate of 72 beats/min (1.2 beats/s), for trial 1 (Fig. 2A), the measured systolic pressure would be 2.5 mm Hg below true systolic pressure. If the cuff deflation rate were 5 mm Hg/s (trial 2), the error would be 4.2 mm Hg. If the heart rate is slower, the error would be larger. The same logic can be applied to the identification of diastolic pressure. Therefore, the repeated measurement of blood pressure will necessarily produce a range of values, even when blood pressure and heart rate are constant.

Figure 2B illustrates an incremental decrease in cuff pressure that is employed in most measuring instruments that use the oscillometric method. The amplitude of each increment may be a few mm Hg, and the duration of the increment is usually the time required to detect 2 oscillations in cuff pressure, i.e., 2 heart beats. Therefore, for a heart rate of 72 beats/min, and a blood pressure of 120/80, and using 3 mm Hg increments, it would require 22.1 s for cuff pressure to scan the range from 120 to 80 mm Hg. The sampling time is longer in practice because the cuff if inflated to typically 200 mm Hg, and is deflated to below diastolic pressure.

Cuff Size

All noninvasive methods of measuring blood pressure employ an air-inflated bladder in a cuff to occlude an underlying artery. The function of the cuff is to transmit the counterpressure therein to the underlying artery. The counterpressure is gradually reduced from suprasystolic pressure, and various strategies are used to identify the instant when cuff pressure passes through systolic, mean, and diastolic pressures. Usually the arm or the leg is the site for measurement. Figure 3 illustrates a cuff on the upper arm. Two tubes communicate with the bladder in the cuff. One tube is used to inflate and deflate the bladder; the other tube is used to measure the bladder pressure. It is unwise to use a cuff with a single tube because of the error caused by the pressure drop along the tube during cuff deflation. However, if the pressure gauge is at the cuff, this error is minimized.

The width of the cuff is that dimension measured along the member (Fig. 3). The length is typically twice the width. Nowadays, a Velcro patch is used to lock the ends of the cuff after it has been applied. Importantly, the width of the cuff, in relation to the member circumference, affects the accuracy attainable, irrespective of the method used to measure the pressure. This fact became obvious when blood pressure was measured on infants, children, and obese subjects. It hardly need be stated that the intervening muscles must be relaxed for effective communication of cuff pressure to the underlying artery. Failure to achieve muscular relaxation will result in a falsely high measured pressure.

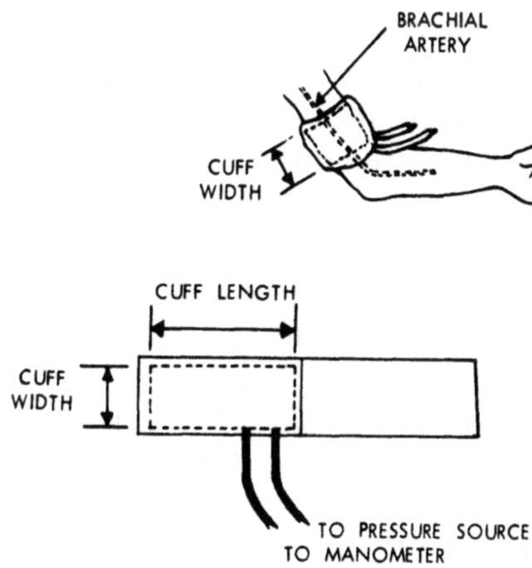

Fig. 3. The blood-pressure cuff.

The first study designed to identify the proper cuff width for the adult arm was conducted by Von Recklinghausen (1901), who used the palpatory method. He found that a cuff width of 10–12 cm was adequate to transmit the counterpressure evenly to the underlying brachial artery in an adult. Since then, the subject of cuff size has received considerable attention. Three cardiology groups: Barker et al. (1939) in the UK, and Bordley et al. (1967,1980) and Kirkendall et al. (1967, 1980) in the US, have made recommendations; the 1967 report stated that the correct cuff width should be "20 percent wider than the diameter of the arm." Because arm diameter is difficult to measure accurately, this recommendation can be restated in terms of the arm circumference as follows: cuff width should be $1.2/\pi$ times the arm circumference, or about 0.4 times the arm circumference (The 1980 committee adopted this recommendation). For a typical adult arm having a circumference of 30 cm, a cuff that is 12 cm wide is optimal. The consequences of using the incorrect cuff width has received some attention, especially in children. The first to address the problem of measuring blood pressure in children were Woodbury et al. (1938), who recorded pressure directly from the umbilical arteries of 37 newborn babies when measuring systolic pressure by the palpatory method applied to the brachial artery. They found that the standard pediatric cuff (4.5 cm wide) gave falsely low readings, but when a 2.5 cm cuff was used, good agreement was obtained with direct umbilical artery systolic pressure.

Robinow et al. (1939) investigated the relationship between cuff width and arm size in 62 infants and children between the ages of 6 wk and 13 yr. The auscultatory readings obtained with different cuffs (2.5, 4.5, 6.5, 9, and 11 cm) were compared with simultaneous direct arterial pressure measurements taken from the brachial, midaxillary, or radial arteries. Using appearance and muffling of the sounds as end points, they showed a positive correlation between accuracy of systolic pressure and the ratio of cuff width to arm circumference. A linear regression line plotted for their data indicates that the proper width is approx one-half of the arm circumference. They also reported that the cuff width for best agreement with systolic pressure was not necessarily that for optimal agreement with diastolic pressure. Diastolic pressures were usually difficult to obtain, and hence unreliable. They advocated the use of cuffs of three different widths (2.5, 5, and 9 cm.), the smallest for newborn babies, the 5 cm cuff for children 1 yr, and the 9 cm cuff for children 1–13 yr of age. With these cuffs applied to the various age groups, auscultatory systolic pressures were −1, +0.3, and −2.1 mm Hg, respectively. For diastolic pressures with the 5 and 9 cm cuffs, the auscultatory values were 11 and 4.6 mm Hg too high, respectively.

The optimum cuff width for the measurement of systolic pressure in the child's arm was also investigated by Moss and Adams (1965), who measured systolic auscultatory blood pressure using 5,7, 9.5, and 12 cm cuffs applied to the arms of 128 subjects ranging in age from 3 to 19 yr. Direct blood pressure was recorded from the contralateral brachial artery. The large amount of data that they acquired was processed to evaluate the correlation between direct and indirect systolic blood pressure on the basis of age, weight, height, and upper arm circumference. A reasonably good correlation was obtained with each of these factors, and the investigators recommended the use of age as the best indicator for selection of a cuff width. They advocated the 5 cm cuff for children 4–5 yr of age, the 7 cm cuff for the age group 5–8½, the 9.5 cm cuff for the 8½–14½ yr group, and the 12 cm cuff for subjects over 14½ yr of age. The investigators presented a graph that showed the errors to be expected when a cuff of a particular size is used at the extremes of the age group for which it is intended. In general, the error was always less than −6 mm Hg at the lower end of the age group, and less than +6 mm Hg at the upper end. The cuff sizes recommended by Moss and Adams relating to age for the measurement of systolic pressure are in general agreement with the recommendations of the various standardization committees. However, Moss and Adams correctly pointed out that age can only be used as a criterion when the child is of normal proportions, and for underdeveloped and overdeveloped children, a cuff of the appropriate size should be used.

In the adult it has been shown by Day (1939), Ragan and Bordley (1941), Kotte et al. (1944), Pickering et al. (1954), Trout et al. (1956), Orma et al. (1960), Berliner et al. (1961), King (1967) and Kvols et al. (1969) that use of the standard 12 cm wide cuff gives falsely high values for pressure when applied to large arms.

Ragan and Bordley (1941) used the appearance and muffling (fading) as the systolic and diastolic end points, respectively. Pickering (1955) summarized their data in a table that showed the correction to be added or subtracted to the values obtained when the standard 13 cm cuff was used on subjects with arm circumferences extending from 15 to 49 cm. The pressure obtained after the correction is applied is true arterial pressure.

The relationship between cuff width and size of the member to which it is applied was investigated again by Kotte et al. (1944). By direct measurement of femoral artery pressure, they showed that the 12 cm cuff, when applied to the leg, gave readings that were too high. They advocated use of a cuff 15 ½ cm in width when the auscultatory method is applied to the leg.

Orma et al. (196) described the use of a cuff that is too narrow as "cuff hypertension." It was shown by Trout et al. (1956) and King et al. (1967) that by increasing the arm circumference by wrapping with cotton or sponge rubber, falsely high values for indirect pressure are obtained. Moreover, Neussel et al. (1956) showed that the loose application of a standard cuff to the adult arm provides a falsely high value for indirect blood pressure.

The study of Day (1939) is of interest because it can be repeated easily to demonstrated the effect of cuff width in children and adults. With a standard cuff on one arm and a different size cuff on the other, auscultatory systolic pressure was measured simultaneously by two observers. The arm with the narrow cuff provided a higher systolic pressure. Nowadays we know that it would be necessary to know the pressure in each arm by first making the measurement with two cuffs of the same size.

An interesting Ponderal-Index method of classifying obesity and therefore, identifying the need for a wider cuff was presented by Berliner et al. (1961). They defined the Ponderal Index as the weight in pounds divided by the height in inches. A Ponderal Index greater than 2.817 identifies obesity and the need for a large cuff.

To illustrate the too-wide, too-narrow cuff phenomenon, Geddes and Whistler (1978) measured auscultatory systolic and diastolic pressures of 52 healthy adult subjects, using three standard cuff widths (9, 12, and 18 cm) applied to the upper arm of each subject. The arm circumferences ranged from 21.5 to 36 cm. Figures 4 A, B, C

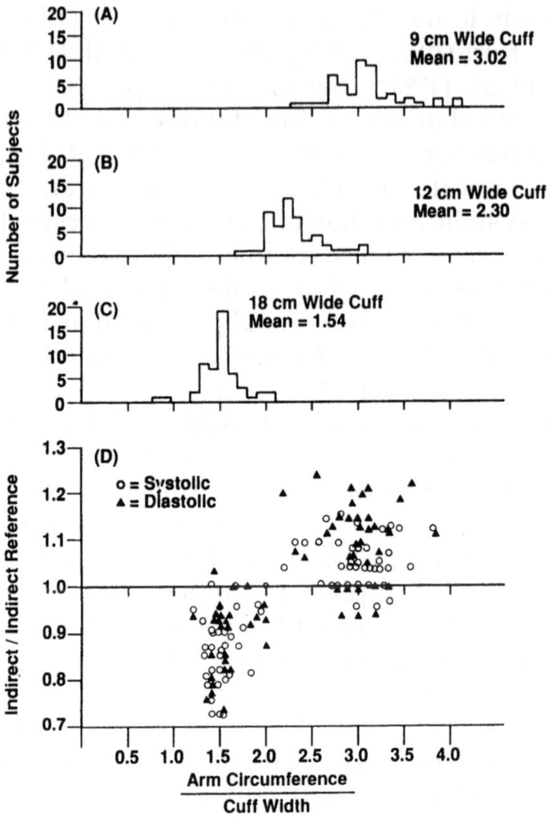

Fig. 4. Number of subjects vs the ratio of arm circumference to cuff width for the 9 cm (A), 12 cm (B) and 18 cm (C) cuff, and the ratio of measured pressure (12 cm cuff) vs the ratio of arm circumference to cuff width (D). (Redrawn from Geddes and Whistler, *Amer. Heart Journ.* 1975, **96(1)**;4–8.)

present histograms showing the number of subjects vs the ratio of arm circumference to cuff width. The appearance and disappearance of sound were used as the end point to identify systolic and diastolic pressures. The values obtained with the 12 cm wide cuff were taken as the reference pressure. The pressure values obtained with the 9 and 18 cm cuffs were expressed as ratios of those obtained with the 12 cm cuff. The pressure ratios were plotted vs the ratio of arm circumference to cuff width. Figure 4D presents the results that demonstrate that when the ratio is slightly less than 2.5, blood pressure is underestimated. When the ratio is greater than about 2.5, blood pressure is overestimated. It is important to observe that, this means that when the cuff width is less than about 1/2.5, or 40% of the arm circumference, blood pressure is overestimated. When the cuff width is greater than 1/2.5, or 40% of the arm circumference, blood pressure is underestimated. Figure 5 illustrates the nature of this relationship, based on the data reported by Geddes and Whistler (1978). It was found in this study (that used the 12 cm cuff values as the reference), and as well as having been found by others, that the optimum cuff width is slightly different for systolic and diastolic pressures. From the foregoing, it is apparent that special attention should be given to the relationship between cuff width and member circumference.

In addition to the width of the bladder in the cuff, its length has received attention by the various AHA committees. The 1939 committee did not specify any particular length; the 1951 and 1967 committees did. The 1951 committee, under the direction of Bordley, recommended "A length of bag sufficient to half-encircle a limb is adequate provided care is taken by the operator to place it on the side of the compressed artery. Some authorities believe that any risk of misapplication should be obviated by use of a bladder that nearly or completely encircles a limb. The 1967 committee reported that "The inflatable bag should be long enough to go half-way wound the limb if care is taken to put it directly over the compressible artery. A bag 30 cm in length which nearly (or completely) encircles the limb obviates any risk of misapplication." At present, many of the cuffs in use measure approx 12 cm in width by 23 cm in length; this length has been chosen as being adequate for compression of the arms of adults of different sizes. Karvonen et al. (1964) measured indirect pressures obtained with a cuff 14 × 40 cm and 12 × 23 cm, and compared the values obtained with directly recorded brachial artery pressure. Cuff pressures for appearance, point of muffling, and disappearance of the Korotkoff sounds were measured. The large cuff yielded systolic pressure values what were 3.0 ± 1.16 mm Hg too low. Using disappearance of the Korotkoff sounds for the diastolic index, the same cuff yielded diastolic pressures that were 1.4 ± 1.26 mm Hg too high. With the smaller cuff (12 × 23 cm), and using the same criteria, the error depended on the position of the cuff. When applied to the biceps, systolic pressure was 0.5 ± 1.71 mm Hg too high, and diastolic pressure was read 7.6 ± 2 mm Hg too high. When applied to the triceps, the small cuff gave systolic pressure readings of 5.5 ± 1.91 mm Hg too high, and the diastolic values were 4.6 ± 2.36 Hg too high. Simpson et al. (1965) investigated the effect of using cuffs wider (14 cm) and longer (35 cm) than those currently in use. Using the appearance and disappearance of sound as the systolic and diastolic indices, and

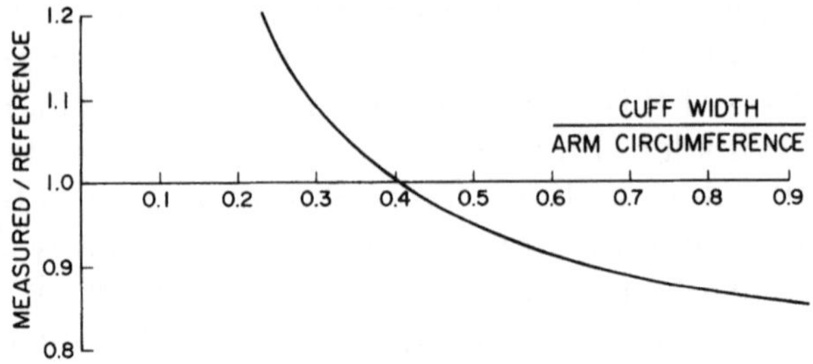

Fig. 5. The ratio of measured pressure to the pressure measured with a 12 cm cuff vs the ratio of cuff width to member circumference. The relationship is for systolic and diastolic auscultatory pressures, measured width a 9,12 (reference) and 18 cm cuff on 52 subjects with arm circumferences ranging from 21.5 to 36 cm. (Curve derived from data published by Geddes and Whistler, *Amer. Heart Journ.* 1978, **96(1)**; (4–8).

comparing the indirect values obtained with those obtained by direct brachial artery cannulation, they found that the indirectly determined pressures were lower than those obtained with the standard size cuff (12 × 23 cm). They also found that the best correlation was obtained with a bladder 12 × 35 cm.

Orma et al. (1960), King (1962), Karvonen (1962), Simpson et al. (1965), and Steinfeld et al. (1974) advocated the use of a longer, rather than a wider bladder in the cuff. They reasoned that a long bladder would allow better transmission of the pressure in the bladder to the underlying artery. However, widespread support for this suggestion has not been forthcoming. At present, the length of the bladder is such that it encompasses about one-half of the member circumference. The 1980 committee chaired by Kirkendall did much to clarify the issue. Table 2 is a summary of the committee's recommendations.

It is useful to recognize that it is the task of the cuff to transmit its pressure to the underlying artery. To do so effectively, any intervening muscles must be relaxed. Contracted muscles will inhibit the transmission of cuff pressure and result in an overestimation of indirect pressure.

Cuff Location and Body Position

The indirect pressure measured depends on the location of the cuff and the position of the body. The traditional location for the cuff is on the left upper arm, as shown in Fig. 3. This site is recommended because the measured pressure is at the level of the left ventricle. If

Table 2
Recommended Bladder Dimensions for Blood Pressure Cuff

Arm circumference at midpoint[a] (cm)	Cuff name	Bladder width (cm)	Bladder length (cm)
5–7.5	Newborn	3	5
7.5–13	Infant	5	8
13–20	Child	8	13
17–26	Small Adult	11	17
24–32	Adult	13	24
32–42	Large Adult	17	32
42–50[b]	Thigh	20	42

[a]Midpoint of arm is defined as half the distance from the acromion to the olecranon.

[b]In persons with very large limbs, the indirect blood pressure should be measured in the leg or forearm.

the cuff is placed on the ankle (Fig. 6A), the measured pressure will be higher because of the hydrostatic head of pressure. One foot of vertical distance below the heart adds $12'' \times 25.4\ \text{mm} / 13.56 = 22.4$ mm Hg; one foot of elevation subtracts the same value; Fig. 6B illustrates this fact.

A different situation obtains when indirect pressure is measured on a supine subject, as shown in Fig. 7A. In this case, all arterial measuring sites are at the level of the heart; therefore, there is no hydrostatic head of pressure. However, owing to the differing arterial elasticity at different distances from the left ventricle, the pulse waveform is different, as shown in Fig. 7B. Systolic pressure is higher in arteries more distant from the left ventricle, and the diastolic pressure is slightly lower. The mean pressure decreases only slightly along the aorta, as shown in Fig. 7B. Therefore, it should not be a surprise to measure a higher supine systolic pressure in the leg than in the arm in a supine subject. The diastolic leg pressure is only slightly lower than diastolic arm pressure. The drop in mean pressure along the aorta is small and indicates that the aorta resembles a manifold.

THE PALPATORY METHOD

The palpatory method was the first to be used to measure blood pressure noninvasively: however, it did not gain popularity until

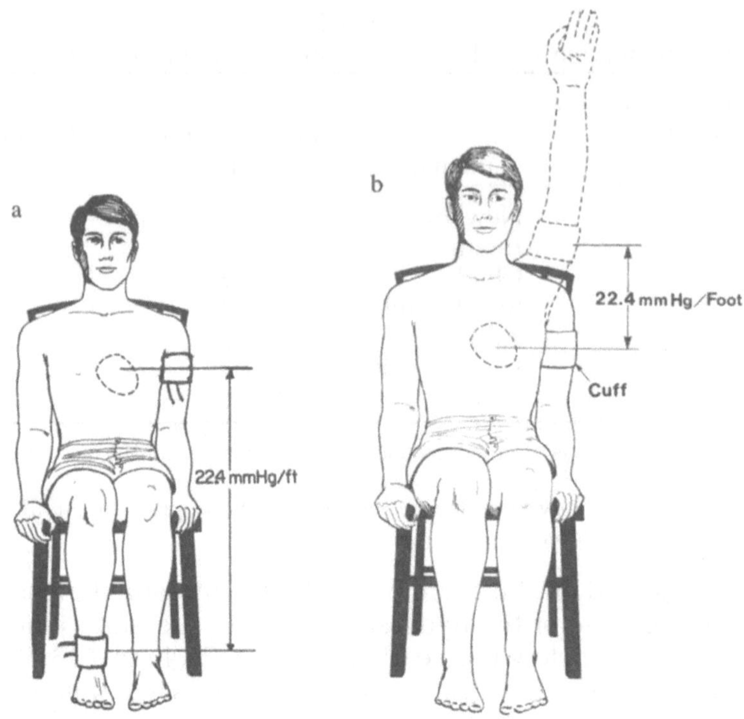

Fig. 6. The importance of cuff location. In A, blood pressure is measured at the ankle, and is falsely high by 22.4 mm Hg per foot of vertical distance from the heart. In B, blood pressure is measured with the arm elevated, and is falsely low by 22.4 mm Hg for each foot of elevation above the heart.

after the member-encircling cuff was introduced at the turn of this century. Although the method only provides an indication of systolic pressure, it retains value because it can be applied when all other indirect methods fail. Typically, the cuff is applied to the upper arm, and the radial artery is palpated as shown in Fig. 8A. The best method of palpation was recommended by Norris (1918), and is shown in Fig. 8B. The palpatory method has been standardized by the AHA (1951), that recommended adoption of the following procedure in conjunction with the use of a cuff having a width that is usually stated as 1.2 times the diameter of the limb, or about 0.4 times the circumference, (i.e., 40% of the arm circumference).

"The patient's radial pulse should be palpated and its rate and regularity estimated and recorded. The pressure of the system [cuff] should be raised to a level about 30 mm Hg above the point at which the radial pulse disappears. Pressure should then be reduced slowly

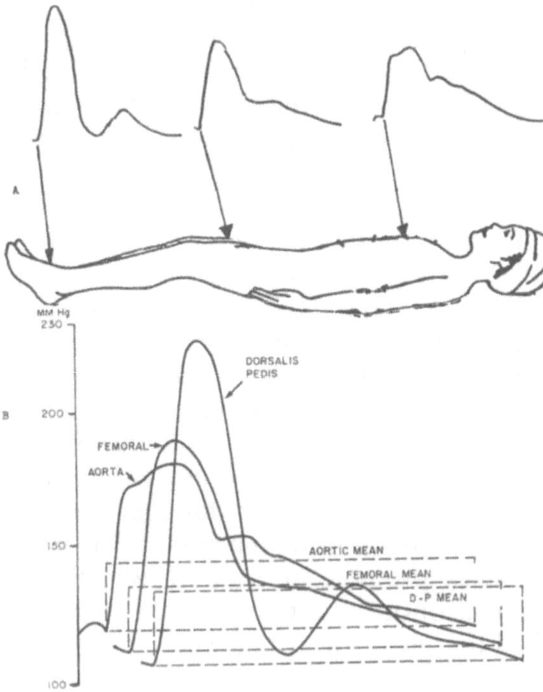

Fig. 7. Arterial pulses at different sites in the supine subject (A) and blood pressure values at these sites (B).

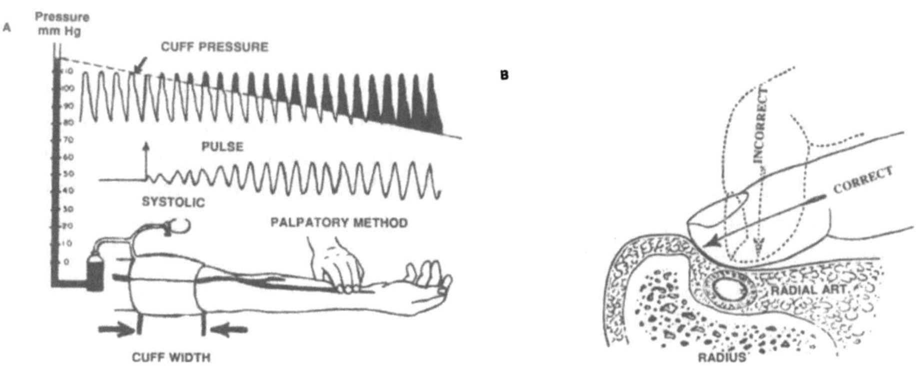

Fig. 8. The palpatory method (A) and technique for palpating the radial artery (B). (B Redrawn from Norris, G. W. *Blood Pressure and Its Clinical Application*, Lea & Febiger, Philadelphia, 1916.)

from the system at such a rate that pressure in the manometer falls about 2 to 3 mm Hg per beat. The return of palpable beats at the normal rate of the heart should be noted as a preliminary estimate of systolic pressure." This means that systolic pressure is read as cuff pressure when the radial pulse first reappears regularly, that corresponds to the minimum systolic pressure during the respiratory cycle."

Accurate measurement of systolic pressure with the palpatory method requires the development of a sensitive tactile sense. One study by Van Bergen et al. (1954) investigated the relationship between systolic pressure recorded directly, and that measured by the palpatory method. Figure 9 summarizes their results, and shows that palpatory systolic pressure was found to be below intra-arterial systolic pressure by about 30 mm Hg at 120 mm Hg. Their data also show a considerable spread to the palpatory-determined pressures.

The availability of small transcutaneous doppler flowmeters has made it easy to measure flow in a superficial artery, such as the radial. These devices produce an audible whistling tone, the frequency of which is proportional to blood-flow velocity. The doppler flowmeter is used to detect the appearance of the distal pulse when cuff pressure falls below systolic pressure.

When graphic recording is available, cuff pressure and the distal pulse can be displayed together. With this method, it is easy to identify return of the pulse during cuff deflation. Figure 10 illustrates the radial pulse detected with a piezoelectric element over the radial artery, using electrical impedance, and with a photoelectric plethysmograph. Note disappearance of the pulse when the cuff is inflated, and reappearance when cuff pressure falls below systolic pressure. There is no consistent indicator in the distal pulse when cuff pressure passes through mean or diastolic pressure.

It is possible to estimate diastolic pressure if, during cuff deflation, the time of appearance of the distal pulse in the cardiac cycle is measured. Geddes et al. (1981) showed that by using the R wave of the ECG, the distal pulse was latest in the cardiac cycle when cuff pressure fell just below systolic pressure. The appearance time became progressively less during cuff deflation, reaching a minimum at diastolic pressure. This relationship has not been exploited to date.

THE FLUSH METHOD

The flush method consists of first rendering a member (e.g., the arm) bloodless by wrapping it tightly with an elastic bandage, start-

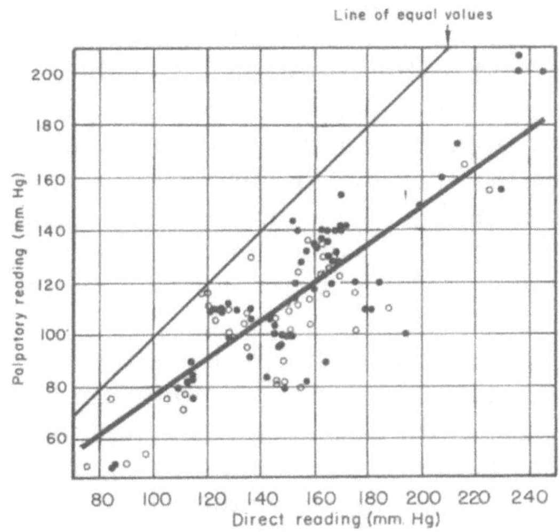

Fig. 9. The relationship between palpatory and direct arterial systoleic pressure. (Redrawn from Van Bergen. F. H. et al, *Circulation* 10; 481–490, 1954).

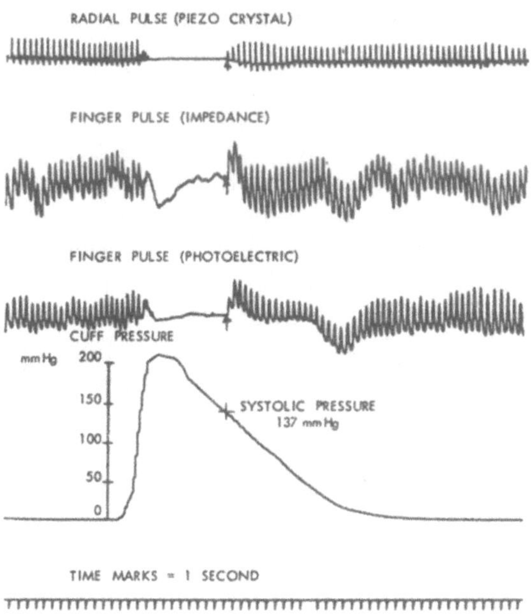

Fig. 10. Graphic recording of the radial pulse, finger pulse (by impedance) and photoplethysmograph, and cuff pressure to determine systolic pressure.

ing at the extremity and progressing toward the torso. Then, a blood pressure cuff is applied and inflated to well above suspected systolic pressure, and held at this pressure when the elastic bandage is removed. Therefore, the member is now bloodless and pale when compared to the opposite member. The cuff is now deflated slowly, and when pressure therein falls just below systolic pressure, the member becomes pink and the subject feels a warm flush. The cuff pressure when blood returns to the member is taken as an estimate of systolic pressure. There is no indicator for mean or diastolic pressure.

Practical application of the flush method was introduced to pediatric practice by Goldring and Wohltmann (1952), who called attention to failure of the auscultatory method in newborn infants. Using the foot or hand as the site for measurement, they rendered the member bloodless by tightly binding it with an elastic bandage, and then applying a pediatric cuff (2.5 cm wide) that was inflated to above suspect systolic pressure. Then, the bandage was removed from the blanched extremity, and it was observed when the cuff pressure was reduced slowly. They reported that "the approximate systolic pressure is the reading at which blood re-enters the foot or hand causing a sudden flush."

Goldring and Wholtmann investigated the relationship between the pressure obtained by the flush method and that obtained with the auscultatory method in a series of older children. Analysis of their data revealed that in the normal children, the systolic pressure obtained by the flush method was on the average 8 (+8 to −14) mm Hg below that obtained by the auscultatory method. In hypertensive children, the flush method was on the average 11 (−7 to −14) mm Hg below the auscultatory systolic values.

Goldring and Wohltmann demonstrated that the method can be applied successfully if the infant is kept quiet by the use of a pacifier or feeding. Good lighting and use of the proper cuff size and a slow rate of deflation of the cuff (not faster than 6–7 mm Hg/s) were stressed.

THE AUSCULTATORY METHOD

Introduction

In a short paper, Korotkoff in 1905 described his method of measuring blood pressure noninvasively in man (*see* translation by Geddes et al., 1966). Employing a Riva Rocci cuff and a child's (Laennec) stethoscope, he described the sequence of sounds that occurred during cuff deflation from above systolic to zero pressure. He stated that the first sound signaled systolic pressure, and the point of disappearance of sound identified diastolic pressure. Figure 11 illustrates the method.

Sound Phases

Because the auscultatory method retains a secure position in clinical medicine, its characteristics, and the phenomena underlying it merit closer scrutiny. When cuff pressure is suddenly raised to above systolic pressure, arterial inflow and venous outflow are arrested. The pressure in the distal arterial segment does not remain at the previous arterial pressure; it falls as blood leaves the distal arterial branches, and enters the capillaries and veins. The Londons (1967) reported that it attains a level of 40–50 mm Hg; others have measured pressures in the distal artery varying between 25 and 50 mm Hg. The venous pressure rises because outflow is occluded. As the cuff pressure is decreased slowly, a stethoscope placed over the distal artery detects a definite sequence of sounds that suddenly appear, change in character, and gradually disappear as shown in Fig. 12. The sequence is so characteristic that several investigators have divided it into distinct phases. Goodman and Howell (1911) recognized five phases. In their own words, the phases are as follows:

1. Phase I—"a loud clear-cut snapping tone."
2. Phase II—"a succession of murmurs."
3. Phase III—"the disappearance of the murmurs and the appearance of a tone resembling to a degree the first phase but less well marked."
4. Phase IV—[the tone] "becomes less clear in quality or dull."
5. Phase V—"the disappearance of all sounds."

Using their values for the pressure "widths" of the four phases in the normal subject, this orderly sequence of events is illustrated in Fig. 12. Although they proposed that the widths of the various phases contained information of diagnostic significance in cardiovascular disease, their proposal has not as yet been validated.

Occasionally, during cuff deflation, the sounds appear, disappear, reappear, then disappear, the first disappearance occurring with a cuff pressure between systolic and diastolic pressures. This phenomenon, known as the auscultatory gap (Fig.12); it was first

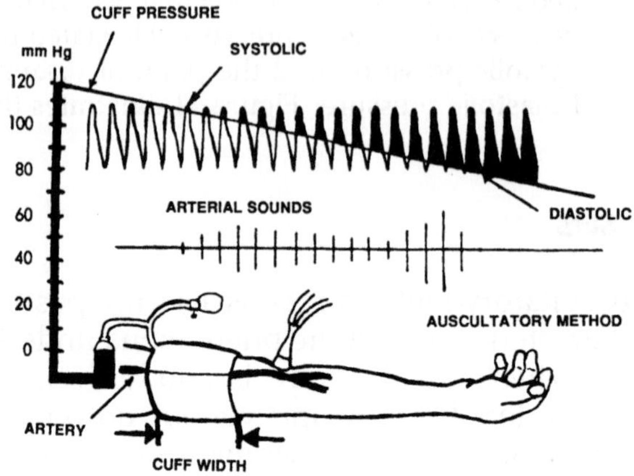

Fig. 11. The auscultatory method of measuring blood pressure noninvasively.

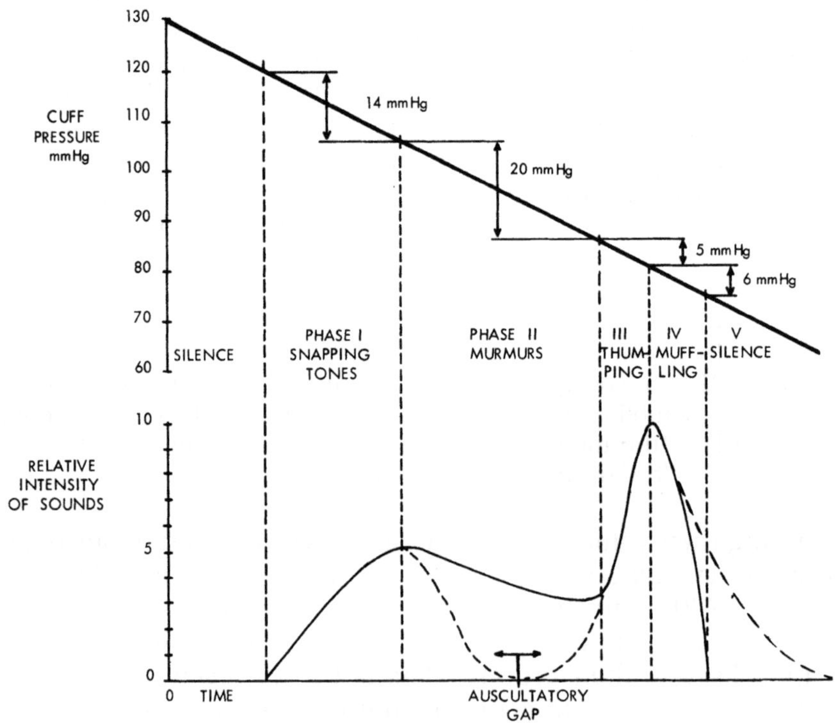

Fig. 12. The five sound phases and their approximate widths in mm Hg, along with an estimate of the intensity of the sounds in the four phases.

described by Cook and Taussig (1917), who reported "In general, the more rapidly the entire estimation [measurement of blood pressure] is made, the less apt one is to meet this period of silence." For some time, the reason for the existence of an auscultatory gap remained a mystery until studies by Berry (1940), and Ragan and Bordley (1941) provided the explanation. The former recalled Sewall's (1940) observation that indicated that auscultatory blood pressure was more difficult to obtain in a standing person, and showed that if, in such circumstances, the subject raised his arm and the cuff was then inflated, and the arm was lowered, the auscultatory sounds were easily obtained. In two patients who exhibited the auscultatory gap, the technique of raising the arm and draining the venous reservoir before inflation of the cuff, permitted obtaining auscultatory sounds without the auscultatory gap. Ragan and Bordley (1941) documented this observation very nicely by presenting records of arterial pressure and cuff pressure, in which the cuff was inflated rapidly and then slowly. In the former case, no auscultatory gap was observed; in the latter, it was. The observations clearly call attention to the importance of a rapid initial inflation of the cuff, and reduction in cuff pressure at a rate adequate to minimize venous congestion in the distal vascular bed.

The Korotkoff sounds, when detected at the antecubital fossa in man, are low-energy acoustic phenomena. In many instances, they are just above the threshold of hearing when monitored with a stethoscope. Therefore, environmental noise can often cause difficulty.

In some subjects, during cuff deflation, the sounds do not disappear after Phase IV (muffling). Instead, they persist to well below diastolic pressure as shown in Fig. 12. This often occurs in young people, and frequently after exercise. Obviously, this event makes it difficult to identify diastolic pressure. To accommodate this situation, it is recommended that three pressures be listed, namely, those for sound appearance, muffling, and disappearance. In other words, 120/90–80 would signfify that, during cuff deflation, the sounds appeared at 120 mm Hg; muffling occurred at 90, and disappearance was at 80 mm Hg. This practice does not improve the ability to identify diastolic pressure. However, listing the three pressures alerts a subsequent observer that the diastolic point is in doubt, thereby perhaps avoiding sending a false signal about an elevated diastolic pressure.

Numerous studies have been carried out to verify the accuracy of the auscultatory method. It should be obvious that cuff pressure must fall just below systolic pressure to obtain the first Korotkoff sound (Fig. 12). Therefore, the auscultatory method must underestimate systolic pressure slightly. The accuracy of the diastolic point is less obvious, because it depends on whether the point of muffling (Phase IV) or silence (Phase V) is used. Not all of the verification studies identified the end point selected, although silence was often preferred. Another important factor is the cuff width in relation to the arm circumference. A target value for the ratio of cuff width to arm circumference is 0.4. Too narrow a cuff results in an overestimation of systolic and diastolic pressures. A cuff that is too wide results in slightly low values. Another cuff-related factor is proper seating of the cuff after application by first inflating and deflating it prior to making a measurement. Failure to do so results in a slightly high pressure for the first measurement. Other cuff-related factors are discussed elsewhere.

TECHNIQUE

The most comprehensive instructions for measuring auscultatory systolic and diastolic pressures have been given by the 1980 AHA Committee, chaired by Kirkendall. Briefly, it is recommended to pay attention to body position, the technique of making the measurement, and reporting details of the method. In summary, the following presents the major points.

Body Position

> "The patient should be comfortably seated, with the arm slightly flexed and with the whole forearm supported at heart level on a smooth surface. Reading taken in any other position should be specified. There is probably no great difference among blood pressures recorded in the supine, sitting, and standing position in normal persons. However, in certain persons there is a striking difference in blood pressure in different positions, and if the patient is in some position besides sitting, this should be noted. When other positions are used, they should be specified with the following abbreviations: L. (lying), St. (standing), Sit. (sitting), R.A. (right arm), L.A. (left arm); i.e. R.A. 148/70, St., L.A. 148/72, L. If the fourth phase (point of muffling of sounds) is used for the diastolic blood pressure, this should be indicated by the value being placed between the systolic and fifth phase (point of disappearance of sound) readings; i.e.

148/78/72/ (78 = fourth phase, 72 = fifth phase). If the sounds are heard to zero, the pressures should be indicated thusly, 148/72/0.

"On the initial examination, one should record the pressure in both arms using abbreviations, i.e. R.A. 140/74; L.A. 152/74. In subsequent examinations, the arm found to have the higher pressure initially should be used.

"The deflated cuff should be applied with the lower margin about 2 1/2 cm above the antecubital space. Care should be taken to insure that the center of the bladder is applied directly over the medial surface of the arm. A preliminary palpatory determination of systolic pressure should be done to give the examiner an estimate of the maximal pressure to which the system needs to be elevated in subsequent determinations.

"The bell stethoscope should be applied to the antecubital space over the previously palpated brachial artery. The stethoscope head should be applied firmly, but with as little pressure as possible, and with no space between the skin and the stethoscope. Heavy pressure will distort the artery and produce sounds heard below the diastolic pressure. The stethoscope should not touch clothing or the pressure cuff.

"With the stethoscope in place, the pressure is raised approximately 30 mm Hg above the point at which the radial pulse disappears, and then released at a rate of 2 to 3 mm Hg/ second. Faster or slower deflation will cause systematic errors.

"As the pressure falls, the Korotkoff sounds become audible over the artery below the cuff and pass throughout the four phases as the pressure declines and sounds disappear.

"In some subjects, particularly hypertensive patients, the usual sounds heard over the brachial artery when the cuff pressure is high, disappear as the pressure is reduced and then reappear at a lower level. This early, temporary disappearance of sound is called the auscultatory gap and occurs during the latter part of phase I and phase II. Because this gap may cover a range of 40 mm Hg. one can seriously underestimate the systolic pressure or overestimate the diastolic, unless its presence is excluded by first palpating for disappearance of the radial pulse as the cuff pressure is raised.

When all sounds have disappeared, the cuff should be deflated rapidly and completely. One to two minutes should elapse for the release of blood trapped in the veins before further determinations are made.

Systolic Pressure

"The systolic pressure is the point at which the initial tapping sound is heard. To make certain the sound is not extraneous, one should hear at least two connective beats as the pressure falls. When the palpatory systolic pressure is higher, it should be recorded and noted as systolic pressure. Both systolic and diastolic pressures should be read to the nearest 2 mm Hg mark of the manometer scale or dial.

Diastolic Pressure

"Muffling occurs when the crisp Korotkoff sounds change and represents sudden diminution or disappearance of sound energy at frequencies greater than 60 Hz. The onset of muffling is the fourth phase and should be regarded as the best index of diastolic pressure for children. Numerous studies indicate that muffling occurs at pressures 5 to 10 mm Hg higher than do the direct intra-arterial diastolic pressures (Appendix 1).

"The fifth phase occurs when sounds become inaudible and should be regarded as the best index of diastolic blood pressure in adults. Although the fifth phase usually occurs with cuff pressure near intra-arterial diastolic pressure, it may fall far below intra-arterial diastolic pressure in children and infants, and in adults with hyperkinetic states, such as hyperthroidism, aortic insufficiency or after exercise (Appendix I). Under these conditions, the fourth phase should be utilized as the best index of diastolic blood pressure. The accuracy of determining the fifth phase depends on the efficiency of the stethoscope and the auditory acuity of the observer."

The fourth-phase (D_4), fifth-phase (D_5) diastolic criterion controversy is unresolved. To shed light on the D_4–D_5 difference, Folsom et al. (1984) carried out a study involving 4885 patients with operators trained to make auscultatory blood-pressure measurements. Audiograms were made on all of the observers to assure that auditory acuity was satisfactory. Comparisons were not made with directly measured pressure; the objective of the study was to quantitate the D_4–D_5 pressure difference. The resolution in the study was 2 mm Hg. They found that in two-thirds of the subjects, the D_4–D_5 pressure difference was zero. In 95% of the subjects, the D_4–D_5 pressure difference was less than 10 mm Hg. In a similar study by D'Souza and Irwig (1976) made on 1037 men ranging in age from 45 to 76 yr, they found an average D_4–D_5 difference of 10.1 mm Hg. Likewise, Reid et al. (1966), in a study involving 676 men ranging in age from 40 to 59 yr, found a D_4–D_5 difference of 7.2 mm Hg.

The foregoing clearly shows that in some subjects, the D_4–D_5 difference in pressure is small. The maximum difference appears to be about 10 mm Hg. The investigators who reported the largest difference recommended identifying the criterion used for diastolic pressure, i.e., phase 4 or 5.

As stated earlier in this chapter, it would be wise to log all three end points, e.g., cuff pressure for the first appearance of sound; that for muffling, and that for the disappearance of sound. Adoption of this technique does not improve accuracy; it only improves communication.

Cuff Deflation Rate

It is useful to consider the effect of cuff deflation rate (3mm Hg/s) on the accuracy of systolic and diastolic pressures. Yong and Geddes (1987) conducted a model study in which heart rate could be selected and the effect of cuff-deflation rate on the measured systolic and diastolic pressures could be studied. Figure 13 presents the results and shows that the slower the heart rate, the larger the error in systolic and diastolic pressures. By using a cuff-deflation rate that is based on heart rate, e.g. 3 mm Hg/beat, the accuracy is the same for all heart rates.

Monitoring Site

The downstream site for the loudest Korotkoff sounds has received some attention. The 1980 AHA committee (Kirkendall) recommended that the "bell of the stethoscope should be applied to the antecubital space over the previously palpated brachial artery." This means that the sound-monitoring site is well downstream from the center of the cuff. The first study to investigate the importance of the monitoring site was owing to Erlanger (1921), who found that the loudest sounds were distal to the site of compression. Allen (1923), in attempting to apply the auscultatory method to the dog, found that the sounds could only be heard with the stethoscope placed under the distal edge of the cuff. Bramwell (1940) reported that the distal point for the loudest sounds moved downstream with increasing blood pressure. Currens et al. (1957) and Geddes et al. (1959) detected strong Korotkoff sounds by placing a microphone in a pocket sewn into the distal edge of the cuff. Wallace et al. (1961) placed a phonocatheter in the brachial artery of human subjects, and found that the sounds were only detectable distal to the center of the cuff. Using an elegant circulatory model, Meisner and Rushmer (1963) found that the sounds were minimal over the point of

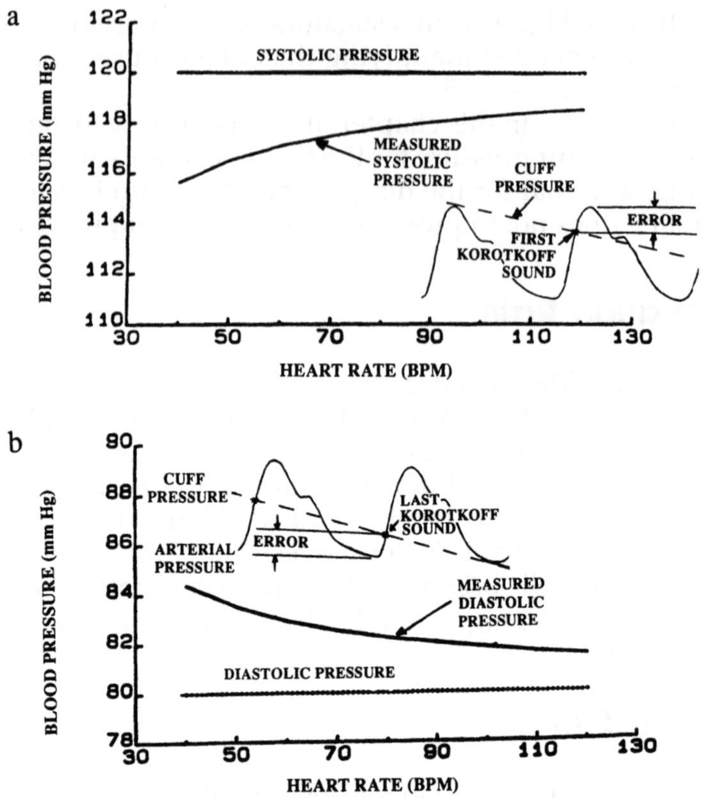

Fig. 13. The relationship between systolic (A) and diastolic (B) pressures and measured systolic and diastolic pressures for various heart rates with a cuff deflation rate of 3 mm Hg/s. (Redrawn from Yong and Geddes, Journ. Clin. Mon. 1987,**3(3)**; 155–159.)

compression, and that fluid disturbances and wall motion did not always accompany each other. They also showed that the velocity of the fluid flow was an important factor in the frequency of the sounds generated. With higher flow, the jet extended further downstream. Collins and Magora 1963) advocated locating the stethoscope receiver at the midpoint of the cuff. Geddes and Moore (1968) obtained loud sounds by mounting a contact microphone to the inner wall of the bladder. The microphone was located at the lower third of the cuff. Many automatic instruments that use the Korotkoff sounds employ a cuff with a microphone in a pocket. The center of the microphone is near the lower edge of the cuff. Although this may not be the optimum site, but sounds can be detected, and with adequate electronic amplification, no difficulty is encountered.

From the foregoing, and recognizing that the events distal to the cuff change considerably during cuff deflation, it is obvious that the optimum monitoring point is not stationary during cuff deflation from above systolic to below diastolic pressure. However, where the optimum site is, and how much it moves during the four sound phases, is not known at present.

Palpation of Korotkoff Sounds

Segall (1940), finding himself without a stethoscope, demonstrated that the vibrations that constitute the Korotkoff sounds can be perceived by palpation. He showed that by palpation of the brachial artery with the thumb (Fig.14), he could feel the vibrations that were ordinarily monitored with the stethoscope. He compared the blood pressure values obtained by the tactile signs and those obtained with the stethoscope. In a series of measurements on 100 patients ranging in age from 2 mo to 86 yr, with systolic pressure ranging from 260 to 80 and diastolic pressures ranging from 120 to 50 mm Hg, the values obtained for both pressures agreed within 2–10 mm Hg by the two methods. This interesting technique may be of value in situations of high ambient noise. It may also be of value to those who find it difficult to hear the Korotkoff sounds. Although it may be difficult to identify systolic and diastolic pressures accurately, mean pressure ought to be easy to identify with Segall's method (*see* next section).

AUSCULTATORY MEAN PRESSURE

Over the years, there have been suggestions that the cuff pressure for the loudest Korotkoff sound identifies mean arterial pressure. For example, Erlanger (1916), when investigating the mechanisms underlying genesis of the Korotkoff sounds in an exposed dog artery, made the first suggestion. Rodbard (1972) stated that the loudest Korotkoff sound occurred when cuff pressure was near mean arterial pressure. To determine the validity of these suggestions, Davis & Geddes (1989, 1990) created an algorithm to quantitate the intensity of each Korotkoff sound. By squaring the amplitudes of the positive and negative waves in each sound complex, and summing these amplitudes, a number is obtained that is proportional to acoustic energy. A plot of the acoustic energy in each

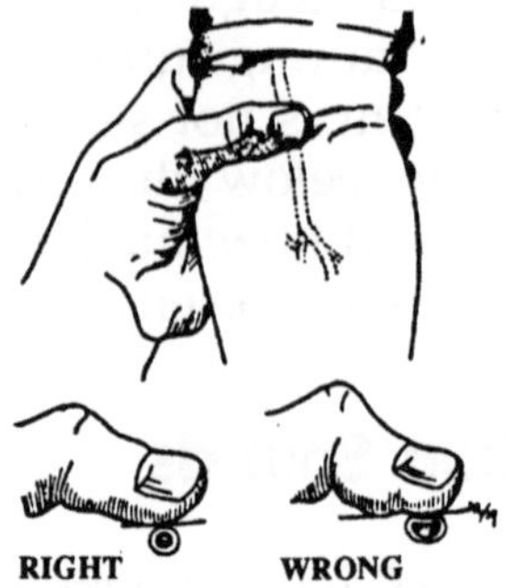

Fig. 14. Segall's method of palpating the brachial artery to identify systolic and diastolic pressures. (From Segall, N. H. *Canad. M.A. J.* **42**; 311–313, 1940, with permission.)

sound complex vs cuff pressure is shown in Fig. 15. Note the similarity of this relationship to the qualitative relationship between relative intensity and cuff pressure shown in Fig. 12 (lower).

In a dog study by Davis and Geddes (1990), it was found that the Korotkoff sound with the maximum acoustic energy provided a pressure slightly in excess of direct mean arterial pressure. In another study in humans (Davis and Geddes 1989), in which the oscillometric method was used to obtain mean pressure, the agreement between cuff pressure for maximum oscillations (mean pressure) and cuff pressure for the Korotkoff the maximum acoustic energy was excellent; the average ratio of the latter to the former was 1.03, with a standard deviation of 0.03.

To date, there has been no human study that compared direct mean arterial pressure and auscultatory mean pressure. However, because the cuff pressure for maximal oscillations has been shown to be in excellent agreement with mean arterial pressure, it is expected that mean pressure obtained, using the auscultatory method, will be accurate.

Synthesis of the Arterial Pulse Upstroke

The Korotkoff sounds are produced when the arterial pressure exceeds the cuff counterpressure and the pulse breaks through. Therefore, the Korotkoff sounds occur during the rising phase of the arterial pulse. Referring to Fig. 16, it is clear that the systolic sound is the latest in the cardiac cycle, and the diastolic sound occurs earliest. This fact was stated by Korns (1926) and used by Rodbard et al. (1957, 1961, 1963, 1965), Ciesielski (1961), and Geddes et al.

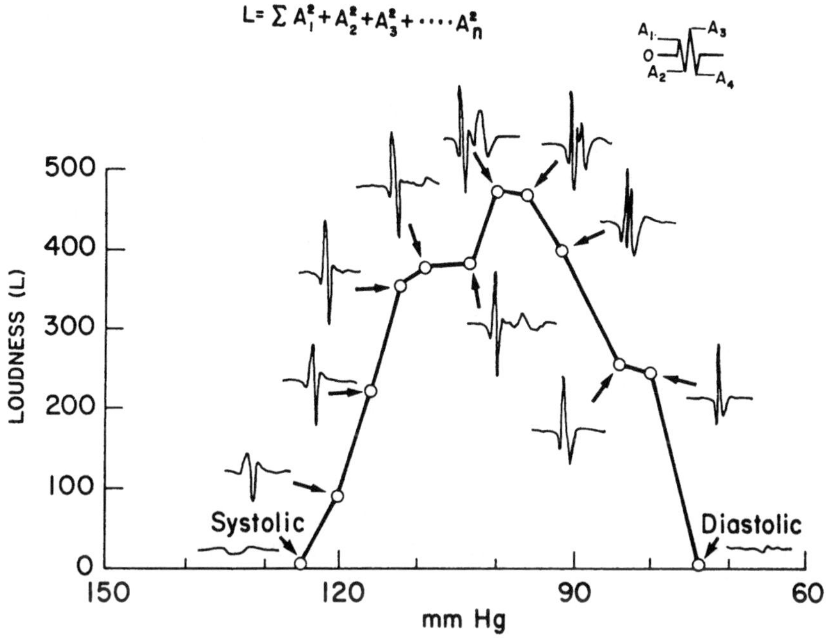

Fig. 15. Auscultatory sound loudness (L) vs cuff pressure. The appearance of sound indicates systolic pressure, the maximum loudness occurs at suspected mean pressure, and the disappearance of sound indicates diastolic pressure. The waveforms identify each auscultatory sound.

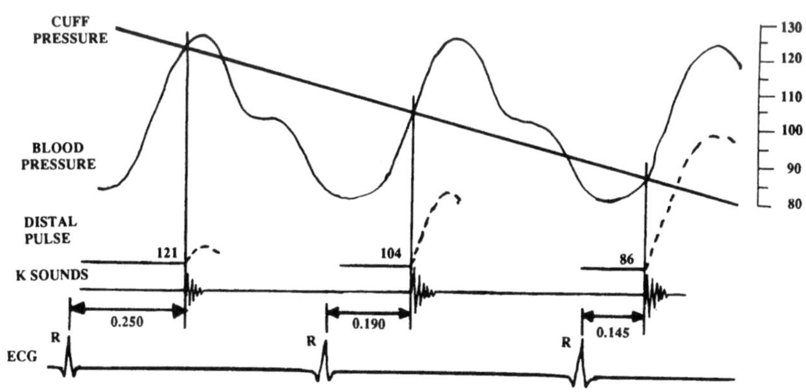

Fig. 16. Principle of arterial upstroke synthesis. The solid diagonal line represents decreasing cuff pressure that intersects arterial pressure earlier in the cardiac cycle as cuff pressure decreases. (Redrawn from Geddes, L. A., et al. *Cardiovas. Res. Center Bull.* 7; 71–78, 1968.)

(1961) to synthesize the upstroke of the arterial pulse noninvasively, and thereby permit calculation of the rate of change of arterial pressure (dP/dt).

The key to using the appearance time of the Korotkoff sounds to synthesize the arterial upstroke lies in using the Q wave of the ECG as a timing reference. A plot of the cuff pressure at which each Korotkoff sound commenced vs the time between the onset of the Q wave of the ECG and the onset of the Korotkoff sound (the Q–K time), displays the rising phase of the pulse wave from diastolic to systolic pressure. Direct arterial cannulation shows (Fig. 17) that the upstroke of the arterial pressure wave is essentially the same as that synthesized using the Korotkoff sounds and cuff pressure.

There are several important times that constitute the Q–K interval. The first is the time required for the left ventricle to develop muscular force. A second is the isovolumic period. The third is the time required for the arterial pulse to travel from the aortic valve to the site where the Korotkoff sounds are detected. This latter, the pulse-transit time decreases with an increase in blood pressure.

The rate of change of pressure (mmHg/s) reflects the vigor of left ventricular contraction and, consequently, contractility. Typical values in a major artery range form 500 to 2000 mm Hg/s. For a time, it was thought that there was a normal value for this quantity, and that deviations would identify cardiovascular disease. Unfortunately, this did not turn out to be so. Nonetheless, it should be recognized that if, in a given subject, the rate of rise of arterial pressure decreases, it is a sign of diminished ventricular dynamics.

Following directly from use of the temporal location of the Korotkoff sounds in the cardiac cycle is the opportunity to improve the estimation of diastolic pressure when the sounds persist to well below diastolic pressure. Observe in Fig. 16 that the sounds get closer in time to the QRS wave of the ECG as cuff pressure decreases. When cuff pressure falls below diastolic pressure, the sounds that may persist will occur no earlier in the cardiac cycle. That, during cuff deflation, the beginning of the upstroke of the arterial pulse does not occur earlier when cuff pressure falls below diastolic pressure was reported by Geddes et al. (1981). Therefore, by using both the intensity of the Korotkoff sounds and their temporal location in the cardiac cycle, it should be possible to obtain a better index of diastolic pressure in those instances when the sounds persist to well below diastolic pressure.

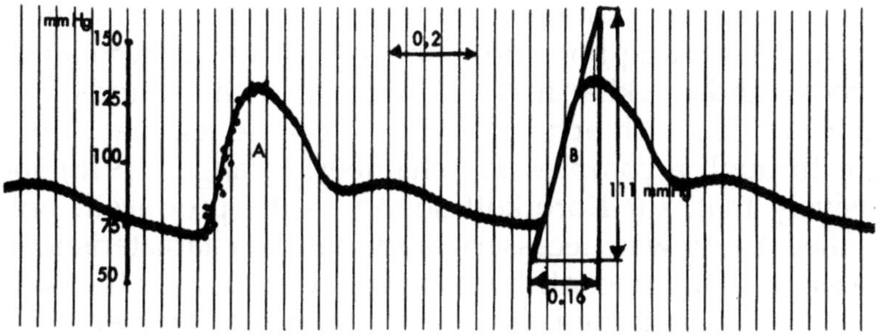

Fig. 17. Synthesis of the rising phase of the arterial pulse wave in the human (A), using cuff pressure and the Q–K time. In B is shown the value for $\Delta P/\Delta T$ = Slope = 111/0.16 = 694 mm Hg/s. (Redrawn from Geddes, L. A., et al. *Cardiovas. Res. Center Bull.* **7**; *71–78, 1968, with permission.)*

GENESIS OF THE KOROTKOFF SOUNDS

Many have speculated on the factors that could produce the Korotkoff sounds; others have carried out studies using models, animals, and human subjects. Despite the complexity of the various factors involved, the origin of the sounds can be attributed to two phenomena. First, those pertaining to the arterial wall, and second, those associated with the flow of blood within the artery (turbulence, vortex shedding, eddy currents, cavitation, and so on.) Because of the relatively low local pressure gradients, cavitation is an unlikely source of Korotkoff sounds. Korotkoff believed that the sounds were caused by the vessel walls and reported "as the wave of blood slips through, the vessel separates and gives a short clapping tone." Gittings (1910) thought that sudden distention of the compressed vessel produced the sounds, but, in addition, the size of the vessel, its accessibility, and the resonating character of the cuff, all contributed to the quality of the sounds. MacWilliam and Melvin (1914) proposed a sudden localized change in shape of the vessel as the originator of the sounds. Flack et al. (1915) conducted a simple experiment that led them to conclude that the Korotkoff sounds have a dual origin—one caused by sudden vessel-wall movement, the other caused by blood flow; this they showed by placing two cuffs on the upper arm of a human subject. The upper cuff was inflated to a pressure of 100 mm Hg to obtain clear Korotkoff sounds. Then, the lower cuff was inflated to well above systolic pressure to arrest the forward flow of blood. They observed that the murmur-like sounds disappeared but the dull sounds persisted, demonstrating both flow and vessel-wall components.

Brooks and Luckhardt (1916) wrote that the sounds "may be due to a nozzle-swish action." When a canine femoral artery was brought through a compression chamber, Erlanger (1916) showed conclusively that, for Korotkoff sounds to be produced, only the blood-filled artery was necessary, and that the characteristics of the compression chamber contributed virtually nothing to the quality of the sounds. He attributed the sounds to water hammer, the noise produced when a flowing stream of fluids is suddenly arrested. In a later study using a similar method, Erlanger (1921) photographed the motion of the arterial wall during decompression and stated that, in addition to the water hammer, an increase in steepness of the pulse front as it passed through the artery being relieved of compression leads to disturbances that produce sound. Edwards and Levine (1952) stated that "murmurs at or distal to the site of compression consist of three components: an early systolic impact, a later systolic stenotic flow and a protodiastolic recoil." Robard and Saiki (1953) proposed that flitter played a role in generating sound. Flitter is the oscillation in the walls of a long, collapsible, fluid-filled tube when the flow exceeds a critical value. Lange et al. (1956) and Lange and Hecht (1958) attributed the Korotkoff sounds solely to "periods of unsteady flow" and stated that a sudden movement of the vessel wall was not needed for production of the Korotkoff sounds. Malcolm (1957) attributed the first and third Korotkoff sound to water hammer and cavitation that produce a forced vibration of the arterial wall; the second Korotkoff sound was attributed to turbulent flow. Kositskii (1958) reviewed the Russian literature on the Korotkoff sounds and stated that "the tones develop as a result of the impact of the portion of blood passing under the cuff on the mass of blood and the arterial wall beyond the cuff. Noises develop in the mass of blood in consequence of the development of an eddying flow." Burns (1959) applied the vortex-generation theory to the development of murmurs in the vascular system; its applicability to the genesis of Korotkoff sounds cannot be doubted. Fruehan (1962) called attention to the fact that vortices can be formed in fluid flowing with Reynold's numbers well below the value for turbulence, and that the shedding of each vortex induces a periodic displacement of the flow pattern. Such a displacement down-stream would be transmitted to the vessel walls. In a plastic tube with a constriction, he showed that the frequency of sounds generated by this phenomenon was directly proportional to the velocity of flow, and inversely proportional to the diameter of the orifice.

Meisner (1962) built a transparent channel through which bentonite-loaded fluid flowed. Bentonite particles allow visualization of the flow pattern when viewed with polarized light. A constriction changed the pattern of flow from laminar to turbulent. A jet formed with its length being proportional to the driving pressure and flow. At the end of the jet, vortices were shed, and persisted for considerable distance downstream. The sounds detected with a microphone placed against the channel were loudest where the vortices were shed.

In a series of experiments on dogs in which high-speed cinefluorograph was used to study flow beyond the occluding cuff, Chungcharoen (1964) reported that the Korotkoff sounds were caused by turbulence alone, and "the vessel wall is not necessary for production of Korotkoff sounds." In an extensive study, in which a hydraulic model was used to simulate cuff occlusion of a brachial artery, Anliker and Raman (1966) postulated that unstable hydraulic amplification occurred owing to local flow disturbances, and several factors (including vessel-wall movement and turbulence) were causative agents. The Londons (1967) believed that the Korotkoff sounds were caused by the vessel walls. One of the most penetrating studies into the mechanism of the genesis of the Korotkoff sounds was presented by McCutcheon and Rushmer (1967), who made photographic studies of the movements of the subclavian artery in a dog as cuff pressure was reduced from systolic to diastolic pressure. Their findings clearly indicated that, as cuff pressure began to approach systeolic pressure, the blood in the artery penetrated nearer and nearer to the center of the cuff. As cuff pressure fell below systolic pressure, "a brief tiny jet could be seen distal to the center of the cuff." As cuff pressure was decreased further, more jets were seen, and the artery appeared partly compressed until cuff pressure was below diastolic pressure.

Because their cineangiograms portrayed only a two-dimensional image of the artery, McCutcheon and Rushmer made casts of canine arteries under various degrees of compression. Examination of the cross-sections of these casts revealed that the compressed arteries were asymmetrically elliptical in shape, and the circumference was reduced by about 50%, when compared to the uncompressed artery. Furthermore, arterial compression produced "fine evenly space, longitudinal wrinkles into the constricted regions." These observations clearly demonstrated the lack of value of model studies using rubber tubes. Such tubes collapse with a constant circumference, and resemble a figure eight when viewed in cross-section.

In the same study, McCutcheon and Rushmer employed two doppler ultrasonic (velocity) flowmeters to study the dynamic events (arterial wall movement and blood flow) that occur during the appearance and disappearance of the Korotkoff sounds. They were able to show clearly that there were two causative factors underlying the genesis of the Korotkoff sounds;

> "1) An acceleration transient produced by an abrupt distention in the arterial wall as a jet of blood surges under the cuff into the distal artery. This produces the first tapping sound which signals systolic pressure. It continues as cuff pressure is decreased and disappears at diastolic pressue.
>
> 2) Turbulent or eddy flow, which follows the initial jet, and produces audible sounds. This factor plays little or no significance in the auscultatory technique."

All of the foregoing suggests a dual origin for the Korotkoff sounds, namely, fluid-flow related and vessel-wall related. It should be recognized that the genesis of the sounds will be different in the four phases; one mechanism predominating in one, and a different one in another. There are, however, other factors that obtain. For example, the rate of rise in pressure (dP/dt) of the arterial upstroke is important (Ehret, 1909, Bramwell, 1926, and Tavel, 1969). A slowly rising upstroke (i.e., a low dP/dt) produces very soft sounds. In fact, this may be part of the explanation for failure of the auscultatory method in hypotension (Rodbard 1962, 1967, Pederson and Vogt, 1973). That fluid velocity plays an important role, dates from the studies by Flack (1915). For the Korotkoff sounds to be audible requires a sufficient flow velocity (Rappaport, 1944, Rodbard, 1953, and McCutcheon, 1967). Interestingly, it has been found that the absence of suspended particles makes the sound louder (Ettinger, 1907 and Goodman, 1911). This suggests that the sounds should be louder in anemic patients. Erlanger (1940) showed that increasing longitudinal stress on the compressed artery reduces the intensity of sounds. Finally, the easiest way to increase the loudness of the Korotkoff sounds is to first drain the venous reservoir by raising the member before inflating the cuff. This technique was described by Berry (1940). The drained venous reservoir results in an increased pulsatile blood flow velocity during cuff deflation, and thereby enhances the sounds. The method is easy to apply, and may be useful in some circumstances.

FREQUENCY SPECTRUM OF THE KOROTKOFF SOUNDS

Beyond an academic interest in the frequency spectrum of the Korotkoff sounds is the need to have this information for the optimal design of automatic devices that use the auscultatory method. In addition, in high noise environments, and with exercising subjects, it is useful to know the minimum bandpass for the sounds for the accurate measurement of systolic and diastolic pressures. The frequency content of the Korotkoff sounds has received considerable attention, and a short review is appropriate.

Among the first to investigate this subject was Korns (1926), who made some 1500 recordings of the auscultatory sounds. In this study, using a membrane manometer, he found sounds with frequencies between 20 and 128 Hz; the frequency of the majority of the sounds was between 40 and 80 Hz. Gilford and Broida (1945) used a band-pass filter having 40% attenuation at 40 and 200 Hz to select only the useful auscultatory information. Geddes et al. (1959, 1962, 1964) studied the frequency spectrum of the normal auscultatory sounds detected by a contact microphone, and reported that although the frequency components occupied a bandwidth extending from 25 to 200 Hz, the major frequency components lay in a band extending from 25 to 80 Hz, with some smaller amplitude components at 100 Hz. Wallace and Khalal (1960) placed a phonocatheter in the brachial artery of humans to detect the intra-arterial sounds, and found small amplitudes with frequencies as high as 600 Hz. In the instrument described by Steen and Grissman (1962), the bandwidth employed was 40–400 Hz. In the NASA project Mercury (1962), the Korotkoff sounds were recorded with a filter centered at 35 Hz. The airborne system developed at the USAF School of Aerospace Medicine (Siahaya et al., 1962, Ware and Kahn, 1963, Kahn et al., 1963), employed a sound spectrum divided into two channels centered at 40 and 100 Hz. It was later separated into three channels peaking at 40, 90, and 150 Hz (Ware and Kahn, 1963). Studies under conditions of flight in which the environmental noise level was high (and, in part, dictated the choice of the filters used) revealed that with the three channels, it was always possible to identify the Korotkoff sounds in at least one of the channels. In a study using the same instrumentation, Roman et al. (1964) reported that satisfactory detection of the sounds could be obtained with a single-channel filter peaking at 100 Hz.

Only a few studies have been carried out in which the frequency spectrum of the Korotkoff sounds has been determined with frequency analyzers. Whitcher (1962),using a spectral frequency analyzer that displayed a graph of the intensity and duration of the sinusoidal frequency components, analyzed the Korotkoff sounds. In normal subjects, he found principal frequency components in the range of 16–200 Hz, with the majority of the components low in frequency; only 9.8% of the energy was above 32 Hz.

In athletes, Masuda et al. (1964, 1966) were faced with the problem of isolating the auscultatory sounds from the noise and vibration produced by exercise. In the resting subject, the frequency spectrum extended from 20 to 100 Hz, with the frequency for the largest amplitude components being around 26 Hz. During exercise, the best signal-to-noise ratio was obtained with a filter having its maximum transmission at 89 Hz. They pointed out that the frequency spectrum differs from person to person, and shifts to the higher frequencies during exercise. Like Ware and Kahn (1963), they examined the sounds detected with channels peaking at 30, 50, 100, and 150 Hz, and found that the results obtained with this multichannel filter were essentially not different than those with the 89 Hz filter. Accordingly, they adopted a filter centered at 90 Hz for their blood pressure measuring system.

The papers by Masuda et al. are of special interest. In two exercising subjects, they found the first (systolic) Korotkoff sound to have a frequency spectrum centered around 80 Hz, and just after exercise, a frequency of 60–100 Hz. Five minutes later, the principal frequency had fallen to 50 Hz. The last (diastolic) sound during exercise had a frequency range of 90–100 Hz that fell to 70–100 Hz just after exercise. Five minutes later, the frequency had fallen to 50–70 Hz.

A study by Rauterkus et al. (1966) of the USAF employed the inflight monitoring system described previously to record the Korotkoff sounds on five normal subjects exposed to the stresses of exercise, the tilt table test, aerobatic flight maneuvers, and centrifuge rides. The sounds were analyzed in a frequency range of 5–160 Hz. Averaging techniques were employed to obtain normalized sounds for the four phases. They found that most of the sound energy was located below 50 Hz. For phases I and IV, most of the sound was below 20 Hz. Phases II and III sounds were broadly distributed in the 5–50 Hz range. The analyzing method used by Rauterkus et al. did not permit analysis of the higher frequency Korotkoff sounds. A reevaluation of the data revealed that there was appreciable acoustic energy located at 46, 104, and 150 Hz. Ware and Anderson (1966) described the frequency spectrum of the Korotkoff sounds in the four phases in resting and exercising normal human subjects. The sounds were analyzed in a frequency range extending from 10 to 400 Hz. Phases I and IV were characterized by low frequencies, and phases II and III by higher frequencies. In general, above 50 Hz, the intensity dropped markedly. With exercise, the energy spectrum in all phases moved toward the higher frequencies. In addition, a noticeable peak appeared in the frequency spectrum at 150 Hz. From the graphs published by Ware, the majority of the energy was found to occur around 20 Hz. The components at 100 Hz were present with an energy of approx one-tenth, and the energy present at 200 Hz was only one-hundredth of that at 20 Hz. McCutcheon and Rushmer (1967) showed that the frequency spectrum extended to 180 Hz. The initial (systolic) sound exhibited a spectrum from 60 to 180 Hz without any dominant peak. At diastolic pressure (the phase of muffling) and below, the 60–80 Hz components became markedly attenuated. The sound spectrum just preceding muffling peaked at about 100 Hz. Burton (1967) reported similar data from the point of muffling.

Figure 18 illustrates the power (amplitude squared) of the Korotkoff sounds at different frequencies, for the four phases from data obtained on a young adult at rest. It is obvious that the highest frequency sounds are in phase three; the lowest are in phase two. Thus, it is clear that the frequency content of the Korotkoff sounds is different in the different phases.

From the foregoing, it is obvious that the principal components of the Korotkoff sounds are low in frequency. It must be recognized that each sound is a complex acoustic transient, with its own frequency spectrum. Although the fundamental frequency of each sound is low, it is the harmonic content (overtones) that gives a sound its characteristic quality, and a close inspection of the spectrograms shows that there are high-frequency components present with small amplitudes. Therefore, for faithful reproduction of the auscultatory sounds, it is necessary to provide a bandwidth wider than that necessary to pass only the fundamental frequencies. The sound spectrograms published by Masuda and Endo (1966) for the resting and exercising subject, show that the major frequency components fall in a band extending from about 20 Hz to about 300 Hz. The data presented by McCutcheon and Rushmer (1967) indicate that a frequency response extending to 180 Hz is adequate to identify the change in sound character that occurs at diastolic pressure. It

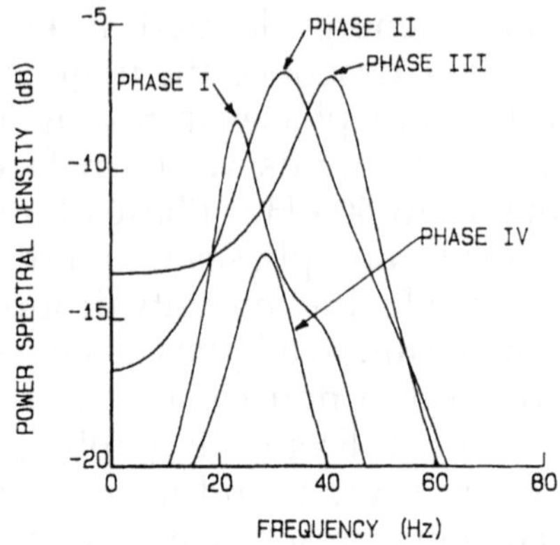

Fig. 18. Power spectra of Phases I, II, III and IV sounds from a resting adult.

would appear that, for high-fidelity reproduction of the Korotkoff sounds, a bandwidth extending from 20 to 300 Hz is required.

It is well known that the auscultatory method fails in hypotensive subjects. One study of the frequency spectrum obtained from such subjects offers a possible explanation. In a series of carefully controlled studies on human subjects. Whitcher et al. (1966, 1967) showed that, with a fall in blood pressure, the sound spectrum shifts to the lower frequencies. In one postoperative hypotensive subject, no appreciable energy could be detected above 8 Hz. When the blood pressure returned to normal, the sound spectrum was in the range of audible frequencies. From this study, it would appear that it is not the auscultatory method that fails in hypotension; it is owing to a failure of the human ear to appreciate low-frequency energy.

Figure 19 illustrates the threshold of hearing at different frequencies, and the estimated intensity of the Korotkoff sounds. This estimate was derived from the data in the papers cited in this chapter.

CHARACTERISTICS OF THE AUSCULTATORY METHOD

The vast amount of epidemiological information includes blood pressure values obtained with the auscultatory method. For this reason, it occupies a central role in medicine, despite the fact that systolic pressure is slightly underestimated, and diastolic pressure bears a variable relationship with directly measured diastolic pressure. The variable relationship is caused by the frequently changed

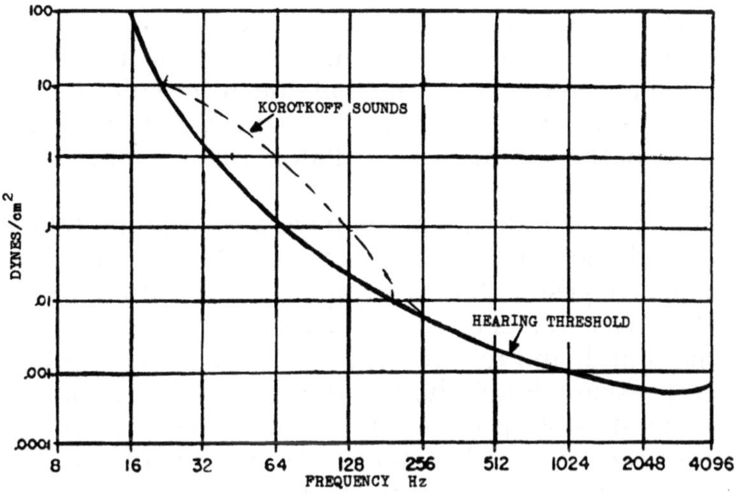

Fig. 19. Threshold of hearing at different frequencies, and estimated intensity of the Korotkoff sounds.

criterion for diastolic pressure. However, listing both phase IV (muffling) and phase V (silence) cuff pressures will do much to remove the uncertainty, but not improve accuracy. Like all of the other occlusive methods, the accuracy depends on use of the correct cuff width in relation to the member to which it is applied.

The Korotkoff sounds are low-energy, low-frequency acoustic events just above the threshold of hearing. Figure 19 illustrates the threshold of hearing and the intensity of the Korotkoff sounds. Therefore, it is necessary to place the stethoscope (or sound detector) at the proper site and listen for the sounds attentively. Because the sounds that identify systolic and diastolic pressures are faint, a quiet environment is needed. Consequently, the auscultatory method is not suited to a noisy environment. However, when the stethoscope is used to acquire the sounds, the ear and the cortex can discriminate the sounds, even when the environment is not quiet. In fact, it is not too difficult to obtain systolic and diastolic pressures on persons exercising on a treadmill.

Variable success attends use of the auscultatory method on ambulatory subjects. Automatic instruments for this purpose employ restricted frequency response to exclude noise. Geddes et al. (1964) employed the R wave of the ECG to open a time window to listen for the Korotkoff sounds at their expected time of occurrence. The time between the R wave and opening the time window includes part of the ventricular excitation time, the isovolumic contraction period, and the pulse-transit time to the site where pressure is measured. The time window must be wide enough to accommodate more than the time for the rising phase of the arterial pulse at the site of measurement. Recall that the Korotkoff sounds only appear during the upstroke of the arterial pulse. R-wave gating is used in some of the automatic auscultatory devices that also acquire the ECG.

Because the Korotkoff sounds have a dual origin (blood flow and vessel-wall motion), it is necessary to inflate the cuff quickly to avoid venous congestion that will impair the flow during cuff deflation. For this reason, it is unwise to raise the cuff pressure just after the systolic sound, and reduce the pressure to obtain a better value for systolic pressure. Similarly, this practice is not recommended to obtain a better diastolic pressure. If venous congestion is suspected, the member can be raised (before inflating the cuff) to drain the venous reservoir. Then, the cuff can be inflated and the member lowered; this practice will increase the intensity of the Korotkoff sounds.

The auscultatory method fails in hypotension and in infants, because the energy spectrum of the vibrations lies below that for human audition. Likewise, the auscultatory method is difficult to apply to small animals. However, some successes have been reported, using newborn or infant cuffs. Wessale et al. (1985) employed a cuff that contained a contact microphone within the bladder to obtain blood pressure in the dog forelimb. With adequate electronic amplification, clear Korotkoff sounds were obtained, and the correlation with directly measured systolic and diastolic pressures was very good.

OSCILLOMETRIC METHOD

Principle

The oscillometric method employs the amplitude of cuff-pressure oscillations to identify systolic, mean, and diastolic pressures. It was introduced by Marey (1876), who placed the hand and forearm in a water-filled chamber, to which a variable counterpressure was applied. The counterpressure for maximum amplitude of oscillations identified that the vessel walls were maximally relieved of tension throughout the cardiac cycle and blood pressure was communicated to the water in the chamber. The same spectrum of oscillations in cuff pressure were seen when the air-inflated cuff was used. For a time, it was thought that the lowest cuff pressure for maximal oscillations was equal to diastolic pressure. This, however, was proven to be incorrect. Posey and Geddes (1969) showed that at the point of maximal oscillations, the counterpressure corresponded to true mean arterial pressure. Although there are no transitions in the spectrum of oscillations in cuff pressure to identify systolic and diastolic pressures, algorithms based on a percentage of the maximum oscillation amplitude are used to identify cuff pressure equivalent to systolic and diastolic pressures.

Figure 20A illustrates the principle underlying the oscillometric method that employs raising the cuff pressure quickly to well above suspected systolic pressure to occlude the underlying artery. Under the upper edge of the cuff, the artery pulsates with blood pressure, and this pulsation is communicated to the upper edge of the cuff via the intervening tissues. Therefore, small-amplitude oscillations appear on the cuff-pressure indicator. Cuff pressure is then reduced slowly (e.g., 3 mm Hg/s) and when it is just below systolic pressure, a spurt of blood passes through the artery under the cuff, and the cuff-pressure oscillations become larger, as shown in Fig. 20B. This transition from small amplitude oscillations (above systolic pressure) to increasing amplitude, was a criterion for reading cuff pressure to obtain systolic pressure; however, this pressure is slightly above systolic pressure. With continued deflation of the cuff, the oscillations increase in amplitude, reach a maximum (m), and then decrease as shown in Fig. 20B. The point of maximum oscillations (m) in cuff pressure identifies mean arterial pressure. There is no indication for the instant when cuff pressure passes diastolic pressure.

The oscillometric method provides an accurate value for mean arterial pressure. That the counterpressure for maximal oscillations represents mean arterial pressure was shown by Posey and Geddes (1969) in studies that used an exteriorized carotid artery in a compression chamber. Blood from a dog flowed through the artery during these studies. Mauck et al. (1980) reported theoretical and experimental studies that support the mean pressure end point. It is possible to derive values for systolic and diastolic pressures as will be described.

There are no consistent transitions in oscillation amplitude to identify systolic and diastolic pressures. Therefore, cuff pressure for a preselected ratio of the maximum amplitude is selected. For systolic pressure, cuff pressure for a ratio of 50% of maximum amplitude is often selected. For diastolic pressure, the ratio is about 80%.

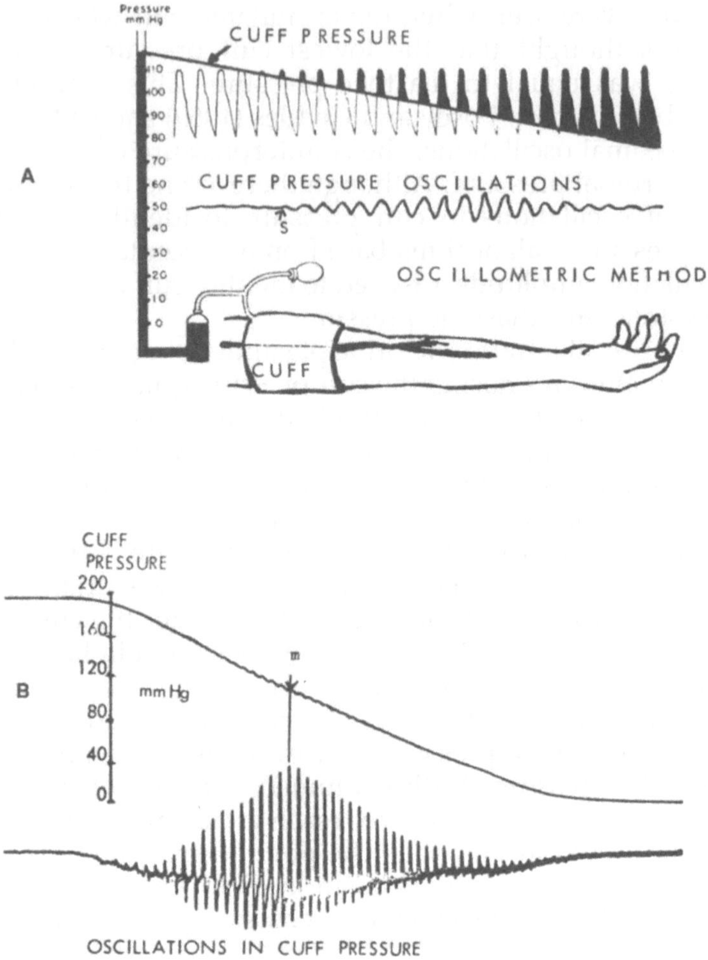

Fig. 20. The oscillometric method (A) and cuff pressure, and amplified cuff-pressure oscillations (B), showing a maximum (m) that corresponds to mean pressure.

To investigate the constancy of the systolic and diastolic criteria, Geddes et al. (1982) carried out studies in adult human subjects, using the auscultatory method as the reference. A standard (12cm) cuff containing a tiny contact microphone within the bladder (Geddes et al. 1968) was applied to the upper arms of 23 subjects. Cuff pressure, along with the Korotkoff sounds and amplified cuff-pressure oscillations, were recorded. The auscultatory sounds were monitored aurally, and the first (Phase I) sound and the point of silence (phase V) were used to indicate systolic and diastolic pressures, respectively. Data were obtained at normal and elevated blood pressures, produced by exercise, followed by isometric contraction of the leg muscles to maintain a high peripheral resistance. Figure 21 illustrates a typical record, and reveals several important features. For example, cuff pressure for systolic oscillometric pressures (S_o), as signaled by the sudden increase in cuff pressure oscillations, was slightly above cuff pressure using the first Korotkoff sound, that identifies auscultatory systolic pressure that is known to be slightly below intra-arterial systolic pressure. At normal systolic pressure (120 mm Hg), this oscillometric criterion overestimated systolic pressure by 8%.

In the same subjects, the amplitude of cuff-pressure oscillations (A_s) that corresponded to auscultatory systolic pressure was measured and expressed as a ratio of the maximum amplitude (A_m), that occurs at mean pressure. For 23 subjects, the ratio of A_s/A_m decreased from 0.57 to 0.45 over the systolic pressure range of 100 to 190 mm Hg. At normal systolic pressure (120 mm Hg), the ratio was 0.55.

The oscillation amplitude (A_d) corresponding to auscultatory diastolic pressure was measured and expressed as a ratio of the maximum amplitude (A_m), that occurs at mean pressure. In the 23 subjects, the ratio of A_d/A_m decreased from 0.82 to 0.74 over the diastolic pressure range of 55 to 115 mm Hg. At normal diastolic pressure (80 mm Hg), the ratio was 0.82.

There are many commercially available instruments that use the oscillometric method to indicate systolic and diastolic pressures. The end points used to identify these pressures are proprietary. Nonetheless, most manufacturers have carried out studies to verify the accuracy of their chosen end points.

Verification studies to confirm that cuff pressure for maximal oscillations identifies arterial pressure in adult subjects were carried out by Ramsey (1979) and Yelderman and Ream (1979), who showed that there is a high correlation between indirectly and directly measured mean blood pressure. Figure 22 presents the data obtained by Ramsey (1979). A similar study was reported by Kimble et al. (1981), who compared indirect mean (Dinamap) arterial pressure with direct umbilical artery mean pressure in seventeen newborn infants ranging in weight from 700–3600g. The ratio of cuff width to arm circumference was between 0.45 and 0.70. The indirect Dinamap (D) mean pressure was related to the direct mean pressure (P) by the relationship $D = 0.822P + 7.48$, with a correlation coefficient of 0.853. The pressure range over which data were acquired was 20–65 mm Hg (mean).

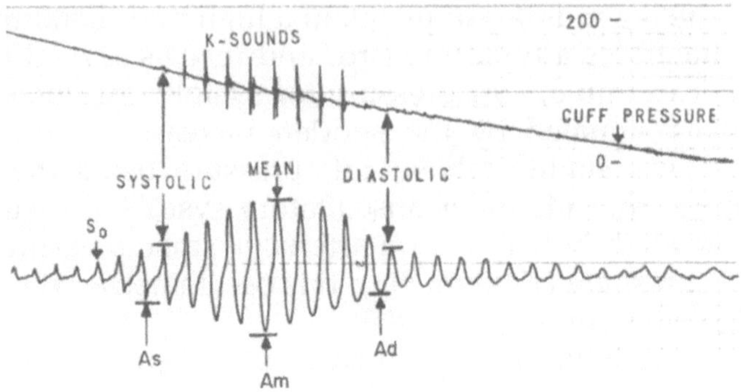

Fig. 21. Cuff pressure with superimposed Korotkoff sounds and amplified cuff-pressure oscillations. S_0 is the point where cuff-pressure oscillations start to increase. A_s is the amplitude corresponding to auscultatory systolic pressure, and A_d is the amplitude corresponding to auscultatory disatolic pressure. A_m is the maximum oscillation amplitude that signals mean pressure.

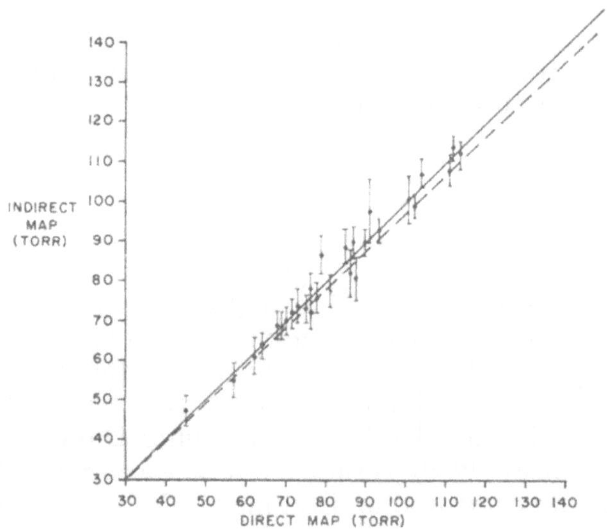

Fig. 22. Indirect mean arterial pressure (MAP) vs direct mean arterial pressure in human subjects, obtained using the oscillometric method. The solid line is a line of equal values, and the dashed line is the regression line idmap = 0.979 (map) + 1.608. The correlation coefficient is 0.98. The vertical lines represent ± ISD. (From Ramsey, M. *Med. Biol. Eng. & Comput.*, 1979, **17,** 11–18 by permission.)

Verification of the algorithms used in the Dinamap (Critikon, Tampa, Florida), was reported by Friesen and Lichter (1981), who compared systolic and diastolic oscillometric pressures with direct arterial pressures (radial, brachial, and umbilical) in premature infants, neonatal, and term babies. Cuff width was chosen on the basis of arm circumference. For systolic pressure, the relationship was $D = 0.94P + 3.53$, where D is the Dinamap reading and P is the direct pressure. For diastolic pressures, $D = 0.98P + 1.70$. These results indicate an excellent agreement between indirect and direct pressures in a patient population in which it is difficult to obtain indirect blood pressure.

Characteristics of the Oscillometric Method

As with the other occlusive methods, the oscillometric method requires use of the proper width for the cuff, in relation to the circumference of the member to which it is applied. Unlike the auscultatory method, blood flow is not required in the underlying artery. The oscillations in cuff pressure are present, with or without blood flow, Posey and Geddes (1969). The end point for mean pressure (maximum cuff pressure oscillations) is definite. An algorithm is needed to estimate systolic and diastolic pressures. Because the only device applied to the subject is a cuff connected to two plastic tubes, the oscillometric method can be used to monitor patients undergoing magnetic resonance or X-ray (CT) imaging. The method is contraindicated in situations when the subject is experiencing vibration, as in exercise.

Shivering also prevents accurate measurement of oscillometric pressures. However, the method is relatively unaffected by audible noise, and is easily applied in such an environment, a typical example being an operating room. Finally, it can be applied equally well to large and small human subjects, and to animals. (Geddes et al., 1977, 1980, and Latshaw et al., 1979).

THE ULTRASOUND METHOD

Principle

There are many ways of using ultrasound to determine blood pressure noninvasively. For example, the transcutaneous Doppler flowmeter can be used to monitor blood flow in a superficial artery when an upstream cuff is used to determine the pressure that arrests blood flow. The range of blood flow velocity in a typical artery, and the choice of an appropriate frequency for the ultrasound, result in an audible signal, the frequency of which identifies flow velocity. When the upstream cuff is inflated to suprasystolic pressure, blood flow ceases and the audible sound disappears. Therefore, use of this method provides only systolic pressure.

Ware and Laenger (1965, 1966) and McCutcheon and Rushmer (1967) described a method whereby ultrasound could be used to measure the pulsatile movements of the brachial artery wall as it was relieved of compression by a pneumatic cuff. They used small flat ultrasound (8 MHz) transmitting and receiving crystals mounted to a piece of Velcro that was placed on the arm before application of the cuff (Fig. 23). With this method, vessel-wall displacement and velocity of movement were obtained, and it was found that the wall velocity (Doppler) signal contained information that identified the instants when the vessel opened and closed as cuff pressure fell below systolic pressure and reached diastolic pressure.

There are many ways of presenting the data acquired by this ultrasonic method. For example, during cuff deflation, when cuff pressure is just below systolic pressure, the vessel opens and then closes when the arterial pulse falls below cuff pressure. Thus, two closely spaced wall-movement signals can be obtained, one for the opening, the other for the closing of the vessel (Fig. 23). As cuff pressure is further reduced, the time between the opening and closing signals increases. Finally, the closing and next opening signal merge and then disappear, because the vessel is open throughout the pulse. This sequence of events is shown in Fig. 23. Therefore, audible monitoring of the opening and closing signals (thumps) during cuff deflation permits easy identification of systolic and diastolic pressures. Electronic detection of these signals can be used to hold cuff pressure indicators at systolic and diastolic pressures. There are commercially available ultrasonic instruments that indicate systolic and diastolic pressures. The methods and algorithms used to identify these pressures are proprietary.

Validation studies using the method of Doppler ultrasound to detect vessel-wall-motion have been reported by Kemmerer et al. (1967), Kardon et at. (1967), Ware and Laenger (1967) Ware et al. (1968), and Stegall et al (1968). Kemmerer et al. compared the systolic and diastolic pressures obtained by the ultrasound method with those obtained by direct cannulation of the carotid artery; they reported that pressures were within a few mm Hg of each other. In

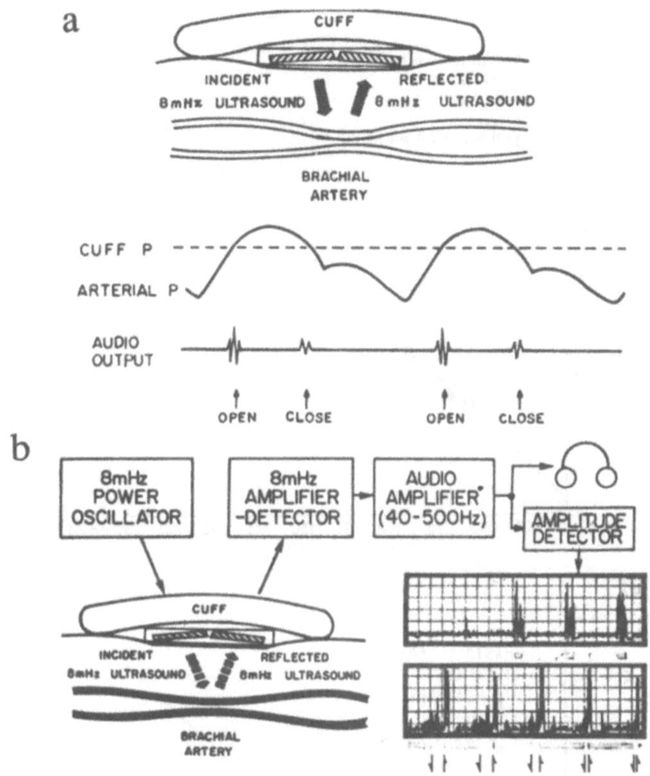

Fig. 23A. Method of using ultrasound to measure vessel-wall movements during inflation of a pneumatic cuff. (From Stegall et al., *J. Appl. Physiol.* **25**, 793–798, 1968, with permission.) B. Changes in the time between artery opening and closing signals during cuff deflation. (From Stegall et al., *J. Appl. Physiol.* **25**, 793–798, 1968, with permission.)

another study, Kardon et al. (1967) obtained similar results in 60 determinations on normotensive subjects. The study by Stegall et al. on 10 normotensive subjects gave an average error in systolic pressure of + 0.1 ± 2.2 mm Hg, and − 0.3 ± 2.1 mm Hg for diastolic. In addition, they were able to identify systolic and diastolic pressures in an extremely noisy environment (± 125 db). In a 51-patient study, Hochberg and Saltzman (1971) compared systolic and diastolic pressures obtained with a commercially available ultrasonic instrument with intra-arterial pressure. In 410 comparisons, indirect systolic pressure (y) was related to intra-arterial pressure (x) by the expression $y = 0.91\chi + 7.4$ mm Hg, with a correlation coefficient of 0.98. Indirect diastolic pressure (y) was related to intra-arterial pressure (x) by the expression $y = 0.92\chi + 6.9$ mm Hg, with a correlation coefficient of 0.91. Figures 24 presents these results.

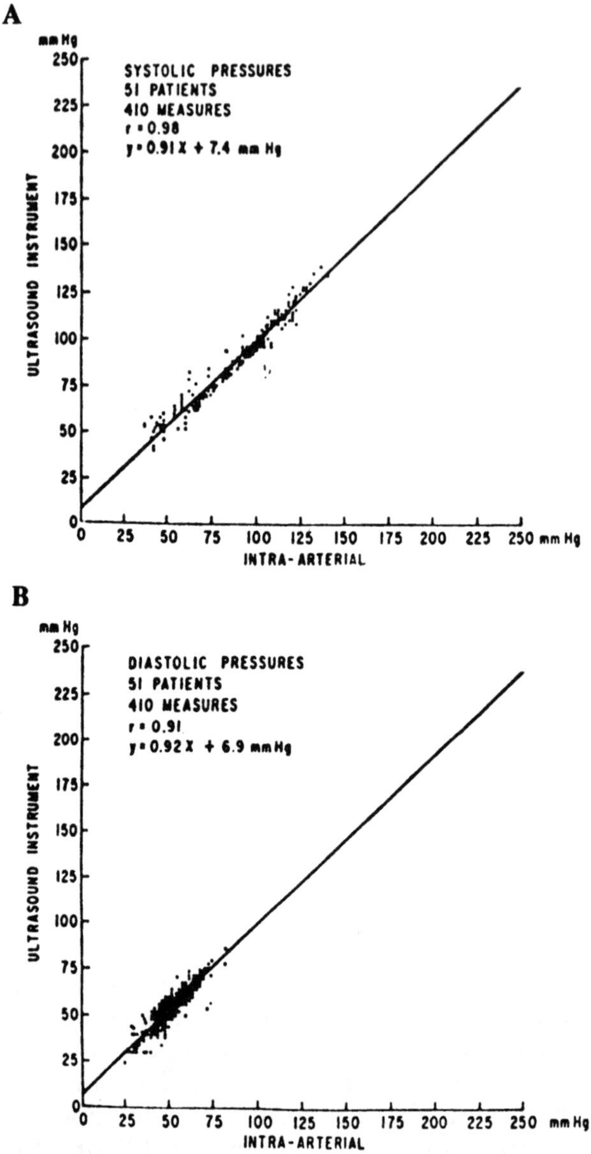

Fig. 24A. Systolic pressures obtained with the ultrasound instrument (BPI) were compared to intra-arterial pressures in 51 patients. The 410 comparisons ranged from 40 to 140 mm Hg, and showed a correlation coefficient of 0.98. The equation of the regression line is y = 0.91 x + 7.4 mm Hg. B. Diastolic pressures obtained with the ultrasound instrument (BPI) were compared to intra-arterial pressures in 51 patients. The 410 comparisons ranged from 25 to 87 mm Hg, and showed a correlation coefficient of 0.91. The equation of the regression line is y = 0.92x + 6.9 mm Hg. From Hochbert and Saltzman. *Current Therap. Res.* 1971, **13**; 129–138, 473–481, and 482–488.

Characteristics of the Ultrasonic Method

To employ the ultrasonic method effectively, it is necessary to establish a good acoustic coupling between the two ultrasonic transducers that are applied to the arm. The transducers (piezoelectric elements) are mounted on the lower edge of the cuff, and coupling is established by placing an ultrasonic coupling gel between the piezoelements and the arm. Two tubes and a cable connect the cuff to the instrument that produces the ultrasonic signals, and displays systolic and diastolic pressures.

Because of the size of the piezoelements, the cuff is slightly bulky, and is best suited to use on adults. The ultrasonic method can be applied to animals, and can be used in high-noise environments, as reported by Stegall et al. (1968). The accuracy is good, as demonstrated by Hochberg and Saltzman (1971); their results are presented in Fig. 24. Despite the good accuracy, the ultrasonic method is less popular today then it was a decade or so ago.

CONTINUOUS NONINVASIVE MEASUREMENT OF BLOOD PRESSURE

Introduction

In psychophysiological studies, inducing polygraphic examinations, it is desirable to detect a change in blood pressure in response to an emotional stimulus. In such studies, a variant of the oscillometric method is employed in which the pressure in a partially inflated cuff is recorded to obtain relative blood pressure. However, the period of observation is limited because the partially inflated cuff soon becomes uncomfortable. The only candidate method that does not require the use of a cuff depends on the velocity of the arterial pulse wave that increases with an increase in blood pressure. Both methods will now be described.

Relative Blood Pressure Method

To identify a change in blood pressure noninvasively, an arm cuff is inflated to a pressure near diastolic, e.g. 80 mm Hg. The pressure in the cuff is recorded continuously with a high-gain, suppressed-zero recoding system. Thus, the recording pen indicates cuff pressure oscillations riding on the cuff-pressure baseline. When the subject is stressed, blood pressure increases, thereby raising the cuff pressure slightly, that is displayed by a rise in the baseline of the recording (Fig. 25A). The oscillations in cuff pressure decrease in amplitude because the rise in blood pressure has moved the point of maximal cuff-pressure oscillations away from cuff pressure. If, however, the cuff pressure had been set to a point just above that for maximum oscillations (mean pressure), an increase in blood pressure results in an increase in cuff-pressure oscillations (Fig. 25B) as well as a rise in the baseline of the recording. This response (Geddes and Newberg, 1977) occurs because blood pressure has moved toward the cuff pressure for maximal oscillations. Therefore, when recording relative blood pressure with a partially inflated member-encircling cuff, an increase in blood pressure causes the baseline of the recorder to rise. Whether the amplitude of the oscillations decreases or increases with an increase in blood pressure depends on the initial setting of the cuff pressure in relation to mean pressure. If cuff pressure is set below the point for maximal oscillations, the oscillation amplitude will decrease; if cuff pressure is set just above the point of maximal oscillations in cuff pressure, an increase in blood pressure will cause a rise in the baseline, and an increase in amplitude of the oscillations. It has not been shown that the rise in baseline cuff pressure is equal to the rise in diastolic or mean blood pressure. The rise in cuff pressure is somewhat less than the rise in blood pressure. Despite the lack of quantification, this change is both reproducible and measurable. It should be obvious, however, that this method can be used for only a short time owing to the discomfort of the partially inflated cuff.

Figure 26 is a record of cuff pressure during a polygraphic examination of a subject suspected of a theft. In such interrogations, irrelevant and relevant questions are asked. All questions are answered with a yes or no. The irrelevant questions establish the response characteristics of the subject. The revelant questions are numbered in Fig. 26.

Pulse Wave Velocity

It has long been known that the velocity of propagation of the arterial pulse from the left ventricle to a peripheral artery is dependent on the dimensions and stiffness (modulus of elasticity) of the intervening vessels. Pulse-wave velocity (c) is defined as the distance that the pulse wave travels in one s. Pulse-wave velocity is

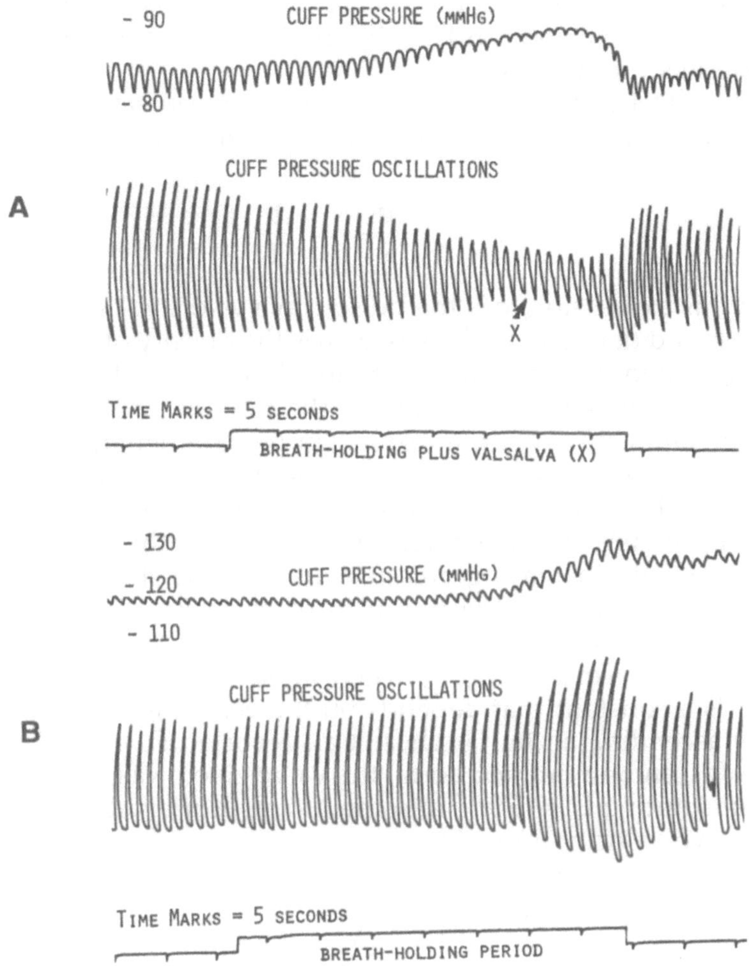

Fig. 25. The "cardiac channel" record of relative blood pressure in polygraphic examination. From *Psychophysiology* 1977, **14**; 198–202. By permission.

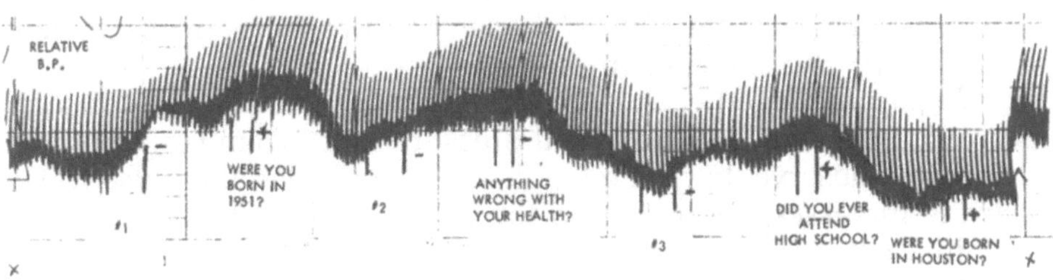

Fig. 26. Cuff pressure during a polygraphic examination. The cuff was initially pressurized to 90 mm Hg and the variations in cuff pressure reflect changes in blood pressure. The relevant questions are numbered.

determined by measuring the transit time (T) between passage of the pressure pulse wave at two different sites along an artery; Fig. 27 illustrates the method.

The velocity of propagation of a pulse wave injected into a thin-walled elastic tube is given by the Moens-Korteweg (1878) equation

$$c = \sqrt{\frac{tE}{\rho d}} = \frac{L}{T}$$

In this expression, c is the pulse-wave velocity, t and d are the thickness and diameter of the vessel, ρ is the density of blood, and E is Young's modulus of elasticity of the arterial wall. The modulus of elasticity of a material is defined as the ratio of stress (deforming force per unit area) to strain (extension per unit length). From the Moens-Korteweg equation, it can be seen that the velocity of propagation will depend on pressure if any of the quantities (d,t,E) depend on pressure. The diameter d increases, and the wall thickness t decreases with increasing pressure. In a 12-dog study, Hughes et al. (1979) showed that the modulus of elasticity (E) of the aorta increases exponentially with increasing pressure (P). The relationship is of the form $E = E_o e^{\alpha P}$, where E_0 is the zero-pressure modulus, α is a constant that depends on the vessel, and e = 2.71828. For the ascending aorta, Hughes et al. reported $E = 667e^{0.017P}$, and for the descending thoracic aorta, the value given was $E = 687e^{0.0016P}$.

Substituting $E = E_o e^{\alpha P}$ into the Moens-Korteweg equation for pulse wave velocity (c) yields

$$c = \frac{L}{T} = \sqrt{\frac{tE_o e^{\alpha P}}{\rho d}}$$

With an increase in pressure, the vessel wall thickness (t) decreases slightly and the diameter (d) increases, indicating that pulse-wave velocity would decrease. However, observe that pressure (P) is the exponent of e, and a slight increase in pressure increases $E_o e^{\alpha P}$ considerably, and overshadows the decrease in wall thickness (t) and increase in diameter (d).

Figure 28 (Pruett el al., 1988) illustrated the in vivo relationship between pulse-wave velocity and pressure for a 30 cm length of the dog aorta. Observe that the relationship is not linear; the pulse wave velocity increases steeply when the pressure exceeds diastolic.

In a practical application, the measurement of pulse-wave velocity requires division of the distance (L) between the two arterial

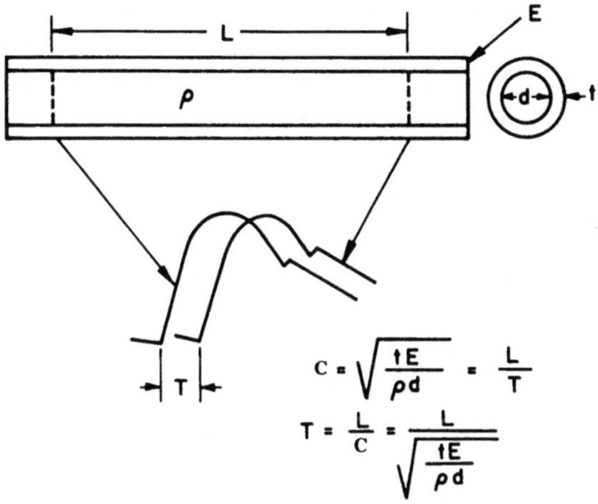

Fig. 27. The propagation time (T) of a pulse along a tube depends on the diameter (d), thickness (t), and modulus of elasticity (E) of the tube. It also depends on the density (p) of the fluid therein, and the length (L) of the tube. c is pulse wave velocity (L/T).

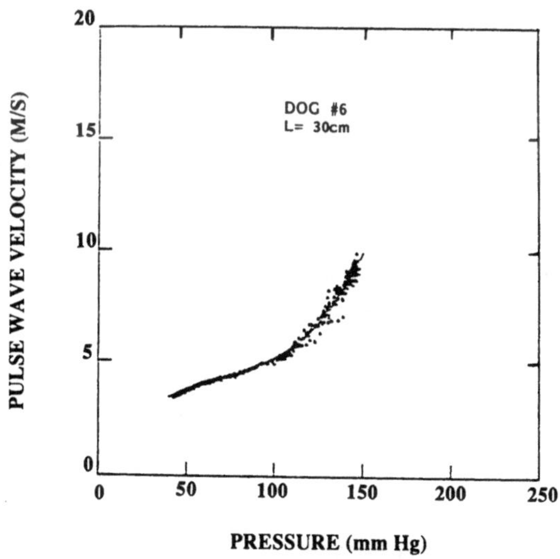

Fig. 28. Pulse wave velocity vs pressure in the dog aorta. The distance between the pressure measuring sites was 30 cm. (Redrawn from Pruett et al. *Ann. Biomed. Eng.* 1988, **16**; 341–347.)

pulse detectors by the difference in time (T) between the start of the upstrokes of both arterial pulses (Fig. 27). The pulse-wave velocity obtained in this manner is the diastolic pulse-wave velocity. To use pulse-wave velocity as an indicator of change in arterial pressure, it is more convenient to measure the change in pulse transit time (T) because the distance between the arterial pulse detectors remains constant. Because pulse-wave velocity is nonlinearly related to blood pressure, the pulse-transit time (T) is also nonlinearly related to blood pressure.

As just shown, pulse-transit time decreases with an increase in blood pressure. Therefore, to use this physical phenomenon optimally, it is necessary to employ two arterial pulse detectors. Many different arterial pulse pickups have been developed (Geddes and Baker, 1975). The most popular pulse detector employs a piezoelectric element that is applied directly to the skin above a superficial artery. Despite the high efficiency of the piezoelectric and other force transducers, there is often difficulty in coupling them to detect the pulse reliably. Even when well applied, it is often difficult to retain them in place for a prolonged period. One simple solution employs a partially inflated finger cot taped to the skin over a superficial artery, and the pressure pulses therein are displayed graphically. Such a technique can be used to detect the brachial, radial, and dorsalis pedis pulses by using cots of a convenient size, applied to the skin over the artery with tape. However, with any of the techniques that apply force to detect the arterial pulse from the skin surface, it should be recognized that the intervening tissue, and perhaps the arterial wall, may become ischemic, and the time of application may be limited for safety reasons.

Despite the century-and-a-half research on the development of a suitable arterial pulse pickup, none exists today that have adequate fidelity to provide the millisecond resolution needed to employ pulse-wave velocity to track changes in blood pressure. Perhaps the use of ultrasound to detect movement of the arterial wall offers the best promise of meeting the requirements for pulse detection.

PRACTICAL APPLICATION

There is an enormous literature on pulse-wave velocity. Pruett et al. (1988) reviewed the literature and described a method of obtaining multiple pulse-transit times from a single pair of arterial pulse waves. Use of this technique has reduced the scatter of data relating pulse wave velocity to pressure (Fig. 28).

When arterial pulse pickups are used, pulse-transit time is measured, but it is difficult to relate this time to pressure. A promising calibration technique was described by Gribbin et al. (1976). Pulse pickups were placed over the brachial and radial arteries, and the pulse-transit time was measured. In order to change the effective blood pressure, the arm was placed in an airtight box to which negative or positive air pressure could be applied. With this technique, the arterial distending pressure could be changed ± 80 mm Hg. At each pressure level, the pulse-wave velocity was measured, and it was demonstrated that pulse-wave velocity increase with an increase in calculated mean arterial pressure.

Another method of estimating the relationship between pulse-transit time (T) and blood pressure can be applied by changing the effective pressure by raising or lowering the member to which the pulse pickups are applied; this method is shown in Fig. 6.

One small point should be recognized, namely, that the Moens-Korteweg equation was developed on the basis of no flow in the elastic tube. Flow along the direction of pulse transmission will shorten the pulse-transit time. However, in the physologic application of pulse-wave velocity, the blood flow is usually much less than the velocity of the arterial pulse wave, and this source of error is usually small.

Attractive as is the pulse-wave velocity method, it is infrequently used, principally because of the lack of suitable high-fidelity arterial pulse pickups, and the need to measure pulse-transit time with millisecond precision. However, the phenomenon rests on a sound physical basis and, undoubtedly, technological advancements will make it more practical.

VASCULAR UNLOADING METHOD

The principle underlying the vascular unloading method was first described by Marey (1876), who placed a hand and forearm in a water-filled chamber that was sealed around the forearm. The pressure in the chamber was recorded when the pressure was raised slowly. With a low counterpressure, small-amplitude oscillations were recorded. As the counterpressure was increased, the oscillations increased in amplitude, reached a maximum, then decreased. Marey stated that, with the counterpressure for maximum amplitude oscillations, the walls of the arteries were maximally relieved of tension throughout the cardiac cycle, and the pressure appearing in the fluid surrounding the arm was equal to blood pressure. In other words, at this counterpressure, systolic and diastolic pressures appeared in the water-filled chamber surrounding the hand and forearm. Much later, it was shown by Posey et al. (1969) that the counterpressure for maximal oscillation was equal to mean blood pressure.

The vascular unloading method was adapted by Yamakoshi et al. (1980) to permit the continuous recording of blood pressure noninvasively in the arteries of a finger. The method used by Yamakoshi and colleages is shown in Fig. 29. To the volar, surface of a finger is placed a photoelectric transducer (PT) that acts as a photoplethysmograph. A light-emitting diode (LED) transilluminates the finger. The finger is placed in the annular fluid-filled, compression chamber (28 mm long and 23 mm diam), that has a translucent sleeve of polyethylene (0.1 mm thick). The fluid in the compression chamber is in communication with a piston connected to an electrically driven actuator. The chamber (cuff) pressure is first raised until the pulsatile oscillations indicated by the photoplethysmograph (PG) are maximal. A closed-loop servosystem employs a position sensor on the actuator, the chamber pressure, and the amplitude of the oscillations in chamber pressure, to keep the fluid-filled chamber at the pressure for maximal oscillations. At this point, the arterial walls are maximally relieved of tension, and blood pressure is communicated to the fluid in the compression chamber. A record of chamber pressure represents pressure in the digital arteries.

Comparison of direct bracheal and digital artery pressure values were made in four normotensive and six hypertensive subjects, as shown in Fig. 30. In commenting on the remarkable accuracy, Yamakoshi et al. stated that "the most important factor in measuring blood pressure by this method is to set the proper reference (REF) value of the servocontrol." They advocated choosing this pressure on the basis of the maximum amplitude of oscillation displayed by the photoplethysmographic record.

Several important facts should be kept in mind when using the vascular unloading method. Perhaps the most important is that the counterpressure is at all times equal to mean arterial pressure. Therefore, perfusion in the member is reduced. No studies have been made in this area; nor is it known how high venous pressure rises in the segment under compression. In subjects with impaired

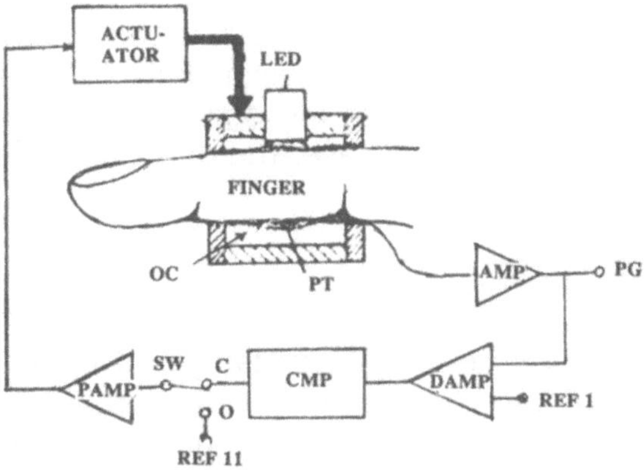

Fig. 29. Equipment employed for use of the vascular unloading method to measure systolic and diastolic pressures continuously. (Redrawn from Yanakoshi, E. et al. *IEEE Trans Bio. Med. Eng.* 1980, **BME 27**, 150–155.)

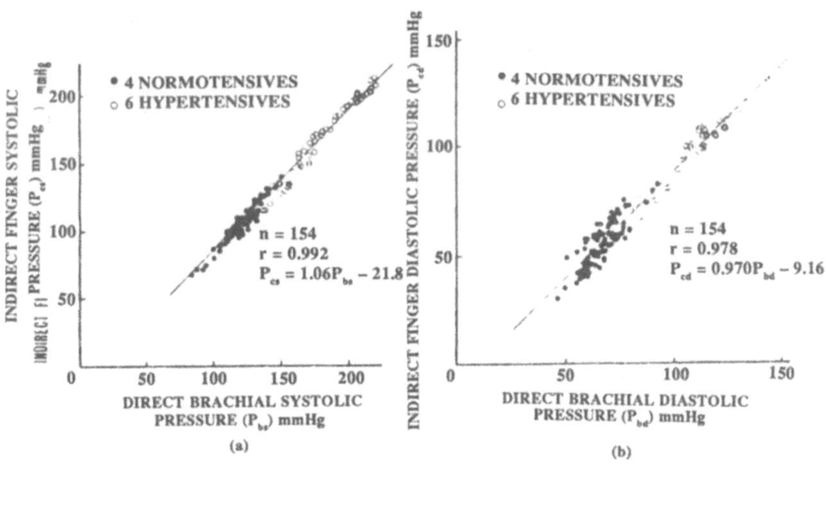

Fig. 30. Comparison of direct and indirect simultaneously measured systolic pressure (A) and diastolic pressure (B) in four normotensive and six hypertensive subjects. Indirect systolic (P_{cs}) and diastolic (P_{cd}) pressures measured by this method are plotted against the corresponding direct systolic (P_{bs}) and diastolic (P_{bd}) pressures recorded by intra-arterial catheters. The solid line in each diagram is the regression line.

circulation, the reduced perfusion may limit the time for safe application of the method. In addition, when the method is applied to the finger, the pressure measured is that in the digital arteries. In all subjects, this pressure is lower than that in the bracheal artery when there is no hydrostatic head between the two sites (Weaver and Bohr, 1950). In thinking about the digital pressure, it is useful to remember that in the typical case, the digits are below the level of the brachial artery.

SURROGATE ARM

Because blood pressure is not constant, and because the indirect methods used in the clinic involve time sampling, it is virtually impossible to determine the accuracy of noninvasive (cuff-based) instruments. To solve this problem, Yong and Geddes (1990) developed a surrogate arm containing an artificial artery sustaining a constant and known pulsatile pressure. The surrogate arm produces all of the phenomena associated with the auscultatory and oscillometric methods of measuring blood pressure.

Figure 31 illustrates the surrogate arm that consists of a silastic sleeve 25 cm long and 30 cm in circumference, clamped to two circular plastic end plates, as shown. The blood pressure cuff is applied to this sleeve when indirect pressure measurement is to be made. Mounted inside is the artificial artery that is surrounded by water with an air space above. The air/water ratio determines the compliance that is adjusted to match that of the human arm. Pulsatile fluid flow is applied to the artificial artery within the arm.

The artificial artery consists of two flat strips of silastic, cemented together at the edges as shown in Fig. 32. When fluid flows throughout the artificial artery, it opens easily. Only a very small excess counterpressure collapses it and arrests flow.

The pressure in the cuff (wrapped around the surrogate arm) is communicated to the artificial artery by the air/water compartment. The Korotkoff sounds, that appear during cuff deflation, are communicated to the cuff microphone by the water at the bottom of the surrogate arm. The cuff is placed so that the microphone is at the bottom of the surrogate arm as shown in Fig. 31. During cuff deflation, the oscillations in the artificial artery are communicated to the cuff. In this way, all of the indicators of systolic, mean, and diastolic pressures are present. Figure 33 shows a graphic record of the pressure in the artificial artery, cuff pressure, Korotkoff sounds, and amplified cuff-pressure oscillations produced by the surrogate arm.

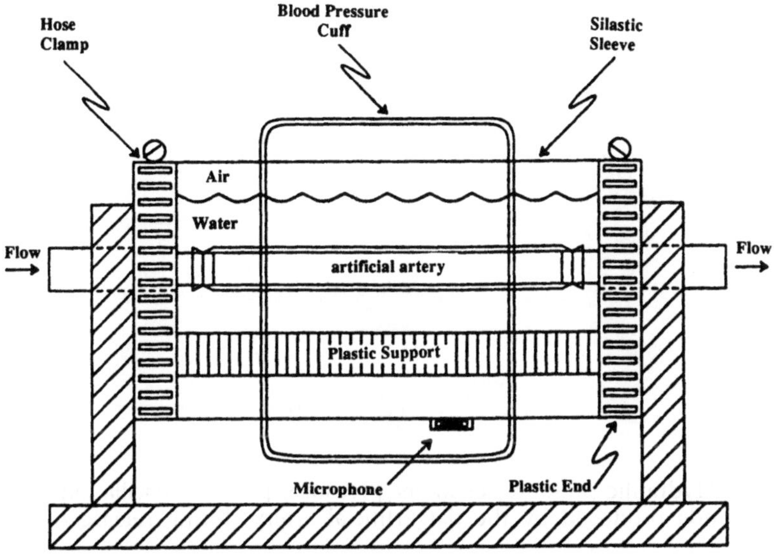

Fig. 31. Schematic diagram of the surrogate arm. Within the silastic sleeve is an artificial artery, a plastic support rod, and an air/water mixture in a ratio that produces an overall compliance equivalent to that of the human arm.

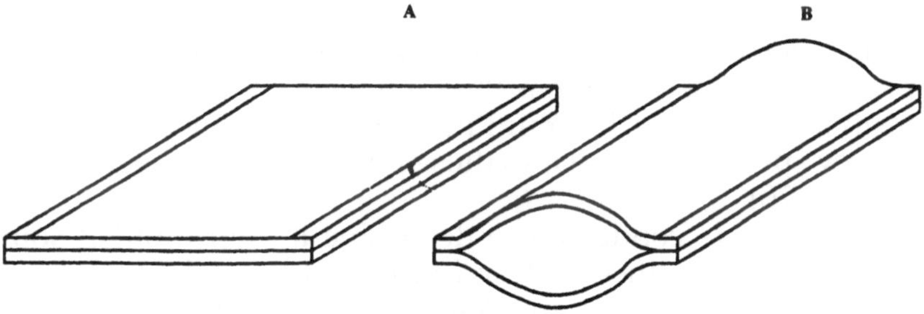

Fig. 32. The artificial artery in its collapsed (A) and expanded state (B).

A hydraulic cardiovascular simulator provides a pulsatile fluid flow with controllable diastolic pressure, pulse pressure, pulse rate, and rate of change of pressure (dP/dt) in the artificial artery. Figure 34 illustrates the essential features of the system. The diastolic pressure is set by the height of the water in the tower (136 cm H_20 = 100 mm Hg). The water is kept at a constant height by a continuous inflow from the water supply. An overflow tube carries away the excess to the drain. Pulsatile pressure is provided by a plastic, water-filled balloon in a sealed box to which intermittent air pressure is delivered via a solenoid valve driven by an oscillator. The air pressure and the duration of its application control the pulse amplitude and the rate of a rise of the pressure (dP/dt). A controlled drain

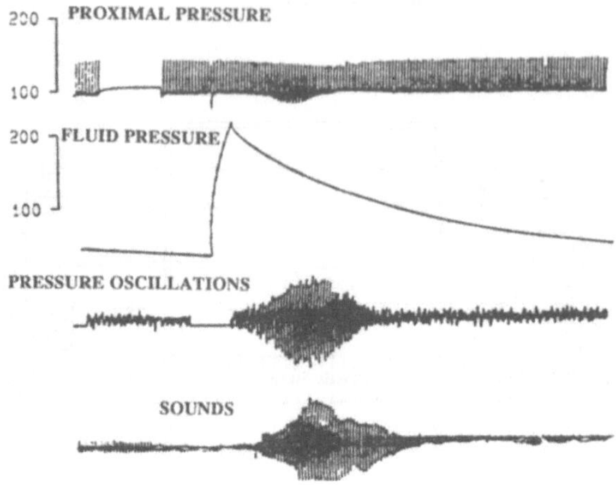

Fig. 33. Hydraulic pressure, chamber pressure, pressure oscillations, and Korotkoff sounds produced by the flat artificial artery during release of counterpressure.

is provided at the inlet to the surrogate arm to keep the pressure at this point constant. By this means, the pressure measured by the pressure transducer (T_1) will be the same if the artificial artery is open or closed during an indirect pressure measurement.

The spectral energy produced by the surrogate arm of phase I (appearance), Phase II (diminished intensity), Phase III (increasing intensity), and Phase IV (muffling) are shown in Fig. 35. These frequency spectra are similar to those reproduced by the human arm (Geddes 1970).

Studies were conducted to determine if the Korotkoff sounds produced by the artificial artery can identify systolic and diastolic pressures. The sounds were detected with a microphone in the lower third of a blood-pressure cuff and monitored, using an audio amplifier connected to a stethoscope-type headset. These endpoints were identified on the graphic record. At the same time, the ability of the point of maximum cuff-pressure oscillations to identify mean pressure was determined using the oscillometric method. Figure 36A shows the correlation between indirect auscultatory systolic pressure and direct systolic pressure. Figure 36B shows the relationship between oscillometric mean pressure and true mean pressure. Note in Fig. 36A, that systolic auscultatory and in Fig. 36B oscillometric mean pressures were accurately demonstrated by the surrogate arm. Figure 37A shows the relationship between Phase IV (muffling) and Phase V (silence) pressure and true diastolic pressure.

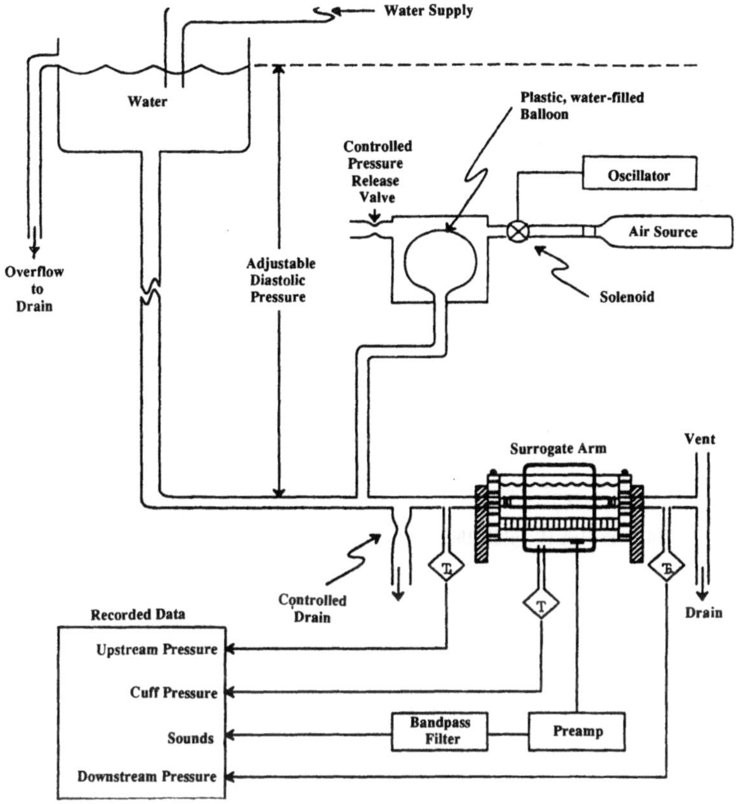

Fig. 34. The hydraulic pumping system (cardiovascular simulator). The height of the water tower establishes a constant diastolic pressure. Pulsatile pressure is produced by the application of pulsatile air pressure via a controlled solenoid valve to the chamber surrounding a plastic water-filled balloon. Pressure applied to the surrogate arm is measured by pressure transducer T_1.

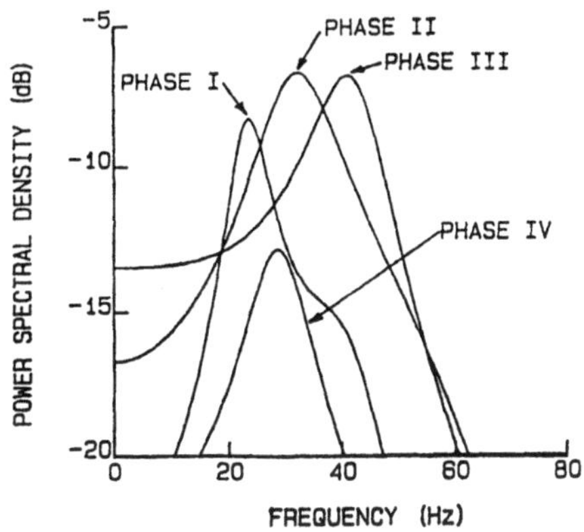

Fig. 35. Composite plots of Phases I, II, III, and IV frequency spectra.

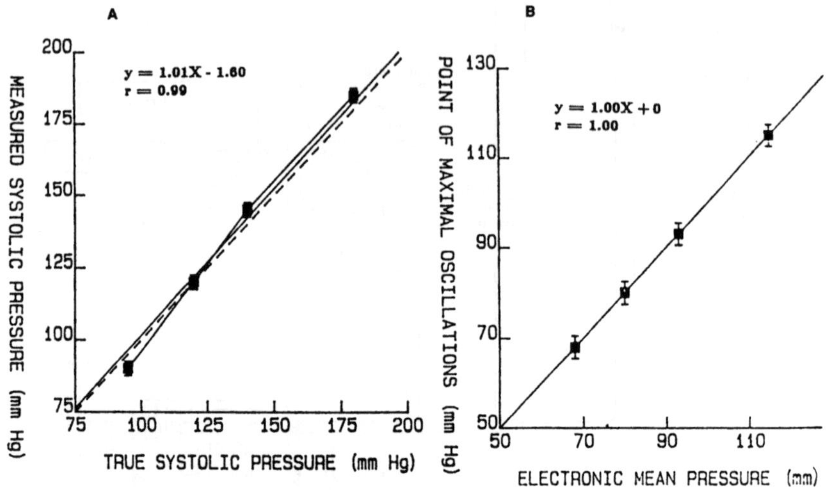

Fig. 36. The relationship between cuff pressure for auscultatory systole (A) and oscillometric mean (B) pressure, and the respective direct pressures. The solid line is the linear regression line, the dashed line is the line of equal values. In both, y is the measured pressure, and X is the true pressure.

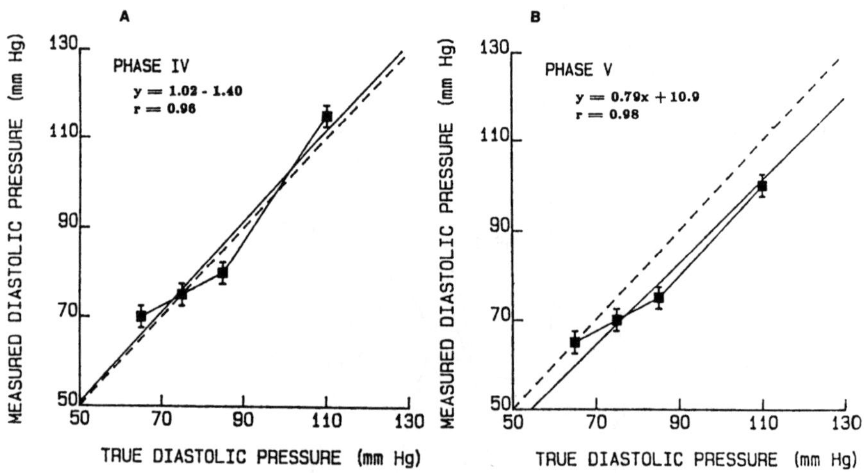

Fig. 37. The relationship between cuff pressure for Phase IV and Phase V Korotkoff sounds and true diastolic pressure. The solid lines are the regression lines; the dashed lines are lines of equal value. Indirect pressure is designated by y, and X is true pressure.

In summary, the surrogate arm is suitable for evaluating the accuracy of noninvasive instruments for measuring blood pressure. In addition, the device can be used as a training tool by those who are learning how to measure blood pressure. It can also be used as an investigative instrument to study the phenomena associated with the auscultatory and oscillometric methods of measuring blood pressure.

REFERENCES

Allen, F. M. Auscultatory estimation of the blood pressure of dogs. *Journ. Metab. Res.* 1923, **4,** 431–443.

American Heart Association: Special Article. Standardization of blood pressure readings. *Am. Heart J.* 1939, **18,** 95–101.

American Heart Association—Bordley, J., Connor, C. A. R., Hamilton, W. F., and Kerr, W. J., *Circulation* 1951, **4,** 503–509.

American Heart Association—Kirkendall, W. M., Burton, A. C., Epstein, F. H., and Freis, E. D. Recommendation for human blood pressure determinations by sphygmomanometers. *Circulation* 1967, **36,** 980–988.

Anliker, M. and Raman K. R. Korotkoff sounds at diastolic pressure—a phenomenon of dynamic instability of fluid filled shells. *Internat. J. Solids Structures* 1966, **2,** 467–491.

Barker, M. H. (and committee). Standardization of blood pressure readings. Joint recommendations of the American Heart Association and the Cardiac Society of Great Britain and Ireland. *American Heart Journal* 1939, **18,** 95–101.

Berliner, K., Fujiy, H., Lee, D. H., Yildiz, M., and Garmer, B. Blood pressure measurements in obese persons. *Amer. Journ. Cardiol.* 1961, **8,** 10–17.

Berry, M. R. Vascular Clinics XII. The mechanism and prevention of impairment of auscultatory sounds during determination of blood pressure of standing patients. *Proc. Staff Meet. Mayo Clin.* 1940, **15,** 699–702.

Bordley, J., Connor, C., Hamilton, W., Kerr, W., Wiggers, C. Recommendations for human blood pressure determinations by sphygmomanometers. *Circulation* 1951, **40,** 503–509.

Bramwell, J. C. Blood pressure and its estimation. *Lancet* 1940, **1,** 138–140 and 184–188.

Bramwell, J. C. and Hickson, S. K. The relation of pulse form to sound production in arteries. Part 2. *Heart* 1926, **13,** 129–151.

Brooks, C., and Luckhardt, A. B. The chief physical mechanisms concerned in clinical methods of measurement of blood pressure. *Am. J. Physiol.* 1916, **40,** 49–74.

Bruns, D. L. A general theory of the causes of murmurs in the cardiovascular system. *Am. J. Med.* 1959, **27,** 360–374.

Burton, A. C. The criterion for diastolic pressure—revolution and counter-revolution. *Circulation* 1967, **36,** 805–809.
Chungcharoen, D. Genesis of the Korotkoff sounds. *Am. J. Physiol.* 1964, **207,** 190–194.
Ciesielski, J. and Rodbard, S. Doubling of the arterial sounds in patients with pulsus bisferiens. *J.A.M.A.* 1961, **175,** 475–477.
Collins, V. M. and Magora, F. Sphygmomanometry, the indirect measurement of blood pressure. *Anesth. Analg.* 1963, **43,** 443–452.
Cook, J. E. and Taussig, A. E. Auscultatory blood pressure determination. J.A.M.A. 1917, **68,** 1088.
Currens, J. H. and Bramwell, G. L. An automatic blood pressure recording machine. *New Engl. Journ. Med.* 1957, **258,** 780–784.
Davis, G. and Geddes, L. A. Auscultatory mean blood pressure. *Journ Clin. Mon.* 1989, 1990, **6(4),** 261–265.
Davis, G. and Geddes, L. A. Comparison of the oscillometric and auscultatory mean blood pressure in man. *Journ Clin. Eng.* 1989, 8(1):15–25.
Day, R. Blood pressure determinations in children. *Journ. Pedi.* 1939, **14,** 148–155.
D'Souza, M. F. and Irwin, L. M. Measurement of blood pressure. *Brit. Med. Journ.* 1970, **4,** 814–815.
Edwards, E. A., and Levine, H. D. Peripheral vascular murmurs. *Arch. Int. Med.* 1952, **90**; 284–300.
Ehret, Ueber Blutdruck und dessen auskultatorische Bestimmungsmethode. Med. Wchnschr. Munchen 1909, **56,** 959.
Erlanger, J. Studies in blood pressure estimation by indirect methods. II. The mechanism of the compression sounds of Korotkoff. *Amer. J. Physiol.* 1916, **40,** 82–125.
Erlanger, J. Studies in blood pressure estimation by indirect methods. III. The movements of the artery under compression during blood pressure determination. *Am. J. Physiol.* 1921, **55,** 84–158.
Erlanger, J. The relation of longitudinal tension of an artery to the pre-anacrotic (break) phenomenon. *Amer. Heart Journ.* 1940, **19,** 398–400.
Ettinger, W. Auskultatorische Methode der Blutdruckbestimmung und ihr praktischer Wert. Wein Klim. Wchnschr. 1907, **20(33),** 992.
Flack, M., Hill, L., and McQueen, J. The measurement of arterial pressure in man. *Proc. Roy. Soc.*, London, 1915, **88 ser. B,** 508–536.
Folsom, A. R., Prineas, R. J., Jacobs, D. R., Luepker, R. V., and Gillu, R. F. Measured differences between fourth and fifth phase diastolic blood pressures in 4885 adults. *Int. Journ. Eped.* 1984, **13(4),** 436–441.
Friesen, R. H. and Lichter, I. L. Indirect measurement of blood pressure in neonates and infants utilizing an automatic noninvasive oscillometric monitor. *Anesth. and Analg.* 1981, **10,** 742–745.
Fruehan, C. T. On the Aeolian theory of cardiovascular murmur generation. *New Physician* 1962, **11,** 433–438.
Geddes, L. A. and Baker, L. E. Principles of Applied Biomedical Instrumentation. 2nd Ed., 1975, John Wiley, New York.

Geddes, L. A., Newberg, D. C. Cuff pressure oscillation in the measurement of relative blood pressure. *Psychophysiology* 1977, **14(2),** 198–202.
Geddes, L. A., Hoff, H. E., and Badger, A. S. Introduction of the auscultatory method of measuring blood pressure—including a translation of Korotkoff's original paper. *Cardiovas. Res. Center Bull.* 1966, **5,** 57–74.
Geddes, L. A. and Whistler, S. J. The error in indirect blood pressure measurement with the incorrect size of cuff. *Amer. Heart Journ.* **96(1),** 4–8, 1978.
Geddes, L. A., Knight, W., Posey, J., and Sutherland, N. Indirect determination of the rate of rise of arterial pressure. *Cardiovas. Res. Center Bull.* 1968, **7,** 71–78.
Geddes, L. A., Voelz, M., Combs, C., Reiner, D. Characterization of the oscillometric method for measuring indirect blood pressure. *Ann. Bio-Med. Eng.* 1983, **10(6),** 271–280.
Geddes, L. A., Spencer, W. A., and Hoff, H. E. Graphic recording of the Korotkoff sounds. *Am. Heart J.* 1959, **57,** 361–370.
Geddes, L. A., Hoff, H. E., Spencer, W. A., and Vallbona. C. Acquisition of physiological data at the bedside. *Am. J. Med. Electronics* 1962, **1,** 62–69.
Geddes, L. A., Hoff, H. E., Vallbona, C., Spencer, W. A., and Canzoneri, J. Numerical indication of indirect systolic and diastolic blood pressures, heart and respiratory rate. *Anesthesiology* 1964, **25,** 861–866.
Geddes, L. A., Combs, W., Denton, W., et al. Indirect mean blood pressure in the dog. *Amer. Journ. Physiol.* (Heart Circ.) 1980, **7,** H664–H666.
Geddes, L. A., Chaffee, V. Whistler, S. J., Bourland, J. D. and Tacker, W. A. Indirect mean blood pressure in the anesthetized pony. *Amer. Journ. Vet. Res.* 1977, **38,** 2055–2057.
Geddes, L. A. The Direct and Indirect Measurement of Blood Pressure. Chicago 1970. Year Book Publishers, 196 pp.
Geddes, L. A., Voelz, M., James, S., and Reiner, D. Pulse wave velocity as a method of obtaining systolic and diastolic pressure indirectly. *Med. Biol. Eng. Comput.* 1981, **19,** 671–672.
Geddes, L. A. and Moore, A. G. The efficient detection of Korotkoff sounds. *Med. Biol. Eng. Comput.* 1968, **6,** 603–609.
Geddes, L. A., Voelz, M., Combs, C., Reiner, D., and Babbs, C. F. Characterization of the oscillometric method for measuring indirect blood pressure. *Ann. Biomed. Eng.* 1982, **10,** 271–280.
Geddes, L. A., Voelz, M., and James, S. Pulse arrival time as a method of obtaining systolic and diastolic pressures indirectly. *Med. Biol. Eng. Comput.* 1981, **19(6),** 671–672.
Gilford, S. R. and Broida, H. P. Physiological monitoring equipment for anesthesia and other uses. *Nat. Bur. Stds. Rep.* **3301,** 1954. Project 1204–20–5512. Supt. of Documents, Washington D. C.
Gittings, J. C. Auscultatory blood-pressure determinations. *Arch. Int. Med.* 1910, **6,** 196–204.
Goldring, D. and Wohltmann, H. Flush method for blood pressure deter-

minations in newborn infants. *J. Pediat.* 1952, **40,** 285–289.

Goodman, E. H. and Howell, A. A. Further clinical studies in the auscultatory method of determining blood pressure. *Am. J. M. Sc.* 1911, **142,** 334–352.

Gribbin, B., Steptoe, A. and Sleight, P. Pulse wave velocity as a measure of blood pressure change. *Psychophysiol.* 1976, **13(1),** 86–90.

Hansen, R. L. and Stuckler, C. G. The "non-hypertension" or "small-cuff" syndrome. *Clin. Pedi.* 1966, **5,** 579–580.

Hochberg, H. M. Automatic indirect blood pressure measurement in multitesting. Tutorial on multitesting. Washington, DC: International Health Evaluation Association, 1971.

Hochberg, H. M. and Saltzman, O. Accuracy of an automatic blood pressure monitor. *Curr. Therap. Res.* 1971, **13(7),** 129–138.

Hughes, D. J., Babbs, C. F., Geddes, L. A., and Bourland, J. D. Measurement of Young's modulus of elasticity of the canine aorta with ultrasound. Ultrasonic Imaging 1979, **1,** 356–367.

Kahn, A., Ware, R., and Siahaya, O. A digital recorder for aerospace biomedical monitoring. *Am. J. Med. Electronics* 1963, **2,** 152–157.

Kardon, M. B., Stegall, H. F., Stone, H. L., Bishop, V. S., Ware, R. W., and Kemmerer, W. T. Indirect measurement of blood pressure using Doppler shifted ultrasound. *Digest of the Internat. Conf. on Med. and Biol. Eng.* (Stockholm: Lungfors Linografiska AB, 1967.

Karvonen, M. H. Effect of sphygmomanometer cuff size on blood pressure measurement. *Bull. WHO* 1962, **27,** 805–808.

Karvonen, M. J., Telivuo, L. J., and Jārvinen, E. J. K. Sphygmomanometer cuff size and the accuracy of indirect measurement of blood pressure. 1964, *Am. J. Cardiol.* **13,** 688–693.

Kemmerer, W. T., Ware, R. W., Stegall, H., and Evans, W. Indirect measurement of human blood pressure by the Doppler ultrasonic technique. *S. Forum* 1967, **18,** 163–165.

Kimble, K. J., Darnall, R. A., Yelderman, M., et al. An automatic oscillometric technique for estimating mean arterial pressure in critically ill neonates. *Anesthesiol.* 1981, **54,** 423–425.

King, G. E. Errors in clinical measurement of blood pressure in obesity. *Clin. Sci.* 1967, **32,** 223–237.

Kirkendall, W. M., Burton, A. C., Epstein, F. H., and Freis, E. D. Recommendations for human blood pressure determinations by sphygmomanometer. *Circulation* 1967, **36,** 980–988.

Kirkendall, W., Feinlieb, M., Fries, E., and Mark, A. Recommendations for human blood pressure determination by sphygmomanometers. American Heart Assn., Dallas TX 1981. *Circulation* 1984, **54,** 1145A–1155A.

Korns, H. M. The nature and time relations of the compression sounds of Korotkoff in man. Am. J. Physiol. 1926, **76,** 247–264.

Korotkoff, N. S. On the subject of methods of measuring blood pressure. *Bull. Imp. Military Med. Acad. St. Petersburg* 1905, **11,** 365–367.

Korteweg, D. J. Ueber die fortpflanzungsgeschwindigkeit die Schalle in elastichen rohren. *Annalen der Physik und Chemie* 1878, **5,** 525–542.

Kositskii, G. I. Theoretical basis for the auditory method of arterial pressure determination. *Sechenov Physiol. J. of the U.S.S.R.* 1958, **44,** 1100–1114.

Kotte, J. H., Iglauer, A., and McGuire, J. Measurements of arterial blood pressure in the arm and leg: Comparison of sphygmomanometric and direct intra-arterial pressures, with special attention to their relationship in aortic regurgitation. *Am. Heart J.* 1944, **28,** 476–490.

Kvols, L. K. Rohlfing, B. M., and Alexandr, J. K. A comparison of intra-arterial and cuff blood pressure measurements in very obese subjects. *Cardiovasc. Res. Ctr. Bull.* 1969, **7,** 118–122, and Personal communication 1975.

Lange, R. L. and Hecht, H. Genesis of pistol-shot and Korotkoff sounds. *Circulation* 1956, **18,** 975–978.

Lange, R. L., Carlisle, R. P., and Hecht, H. Observations on vascular sounds—the pistol-shot sound and the Korotkoff sound. *Circulation* 1956, **13,** 873–883.

Latshaw, H. T., Whistler, S. J., Fessler, J. F., and Geddes, L. A. Indirect measurement of blood pressure in the normotensive and hypotensive horse. *Equine Vet. Journ.* 1979, **11(3),** 191–194.

London, S. B. and London, R. E. Critique of indirect diastolic point. *Arch. Int. Med.* 1967, **119,** 39–49.

London, S. B. and London, R. E. Comparison of indirect pressure measurements (Korotkoff) with simultaneous direct brachial artery pressure distal to the cuff. *Adv. Int. Med.* 1967, **13,** 127–142.

MacWilliam, J. A. and Melvin, G. S. Systolic and diastolic blood pressure estimation, with special reference to the auditory method. *Brit. M. J.* 1914, **1,** 693–697.

Malcolm, J. E. *Blood Pressure Sounds and Their Meanings* (Springfield, IL.: Charles C. Thomas, Publisher, 1957), 93 pp.

Marey, E. J. Physiologie Experimentale. Paris 1876 Masson and Cie.

Marey, E. J. Pressure and speed of blood. Physiologie Experimentale Paris, 1876, vol. 2. G. Masson. Traveaux du Laboratorie de M. Marey. Ecole Practique des Hautes Etudes.

Masuda, M. and Endo, K. Analysis of the Korotkoff sounds before, during, and after the exhausting running. *Bull. Physical Fitness Res. Inst.* 1966, **8,** 187–194.

Masuda, M. and Mihara, T. Automatic indirect determination of arterial blood pressure during exercise. *Bull. Physical Fitness Res. Inst.* 1965, **4,** 25–33.

Mauck, G. B., Smith, C. R., Geddes, L. A., and Bourland, J. D. The meaning of the point of maximum oscillations in cuff pressure in the indirect measurement of blood pressure II. *Journ. Biomech. Eng.* (ASME Trans.) 1980.

McCutcheon, E. P. and Rushmer, R. F. Korotkoff sounds. An experimental critique. *Circulation Res.* 1967, **20,** 149–161.

Meisner, J. E. and Rushmer, R. F. Production of sounds in distensible tubes. *Circ. Res.* 1963, 651–658.

Moens, A. I. Die Pulskurve. Leiden, 1878, E. J. Brill, 147 pp.

Moss, A. J. and Adams, F. H. Auscultatory and intra-arterial pressure. A comparison in children with special reference to cuff width. *Journ. Pedi.* 1967, **66,** 1094–1097.

NASA Project Mercury: Results of the First U. S. Manned Orbital Space Flight, NASA, Feb. 20, 1962. Manned Spacecraft Center. Supt. Documents, Washington, D. C.

Norris, G. W. *Blood Pressure and Its Clinical Application* (Philadelphia: Lea and Febiger, 1916), 424 pp.

Nuessel, W. F. The importance of a tight blood pressure cuff. *Amer. Heart Journ.* 1956, **61,** 905–906.

Orma, E., Karvonen, M. H., and Keys, A. Cuff hypertension. *Lancet* 1960, **2,** 51.

Pederson, R. W., and Vogt, F. B. Korotkoff sounds in hypertension. *Med. Instr.* 1973, **7,** 251–256.

Pickering, G. W. *High Blood Pressure* (New York: Grune and Stratton, Inc., 1955), 547 pp.

Pickering, G. W., Fraser, Roberts, J. A., and Sowry, G. S. C. The aetiology of essential hypertension. The effect of correcting for arm circumference on the growth rate of arterial pressure with age. *Clin. Sci.* 1954, **13,** 267–271.

Posey, J. A., Geddes, L. A., Williams, H., and Moore, A. G. The meaning of the point of maximum oscillations in cuff pressure in the indirect measurement of blood pressure. Part 1. *Cardiovasc. Res. Ctr. Bull.* 1969 **8,**(1):15–25.

Pruett, J., Bourland, J. D., and Geddes, L. A. Measurement of pulse wave velocity using a beat-sampling technique. *Ann. Biomed. Eng.* 1988, **16,** 341–347.

Ragan, C. and Bordley, J. The accuracy of clinical measurements of arterial blood pressure. *Bull. Johns Hopkins Hosp.* 1941, **69,** 504–528.

Ramsey, M. Noninvasive automatic determination of mean arterial pressure. *Med. Biol. Eng. Comput.* 1979, **17,** 11–18.

Rappaport, M. B. and Luisada, A. A. Indirect sphygmomanometry. *Ind. Clin. Med.* 1944, **29,** 638–656.

Rauterkus, T., Feltz, J. F., and Fickes, J. W. Frequency analysis of Korotkov blood pressure sounds using the Fourier transform. *SAM Tech. Rep. SAM-TR-66–8.* USAF School of Aerospace Med. 1966, 46 pp.

Reid, D. H., Holland, W. W., and Humesfelt, S. A cardiovascular survey of British postal workers. *Lancet* 1966, **1,** 614–618.

Robinow, M., Hamilton, W. F., Woodbury, R. A., and Volpitto, P. P. Accuracy of clinical determinations of blood pressure in children. *Amer. Journ. Dis. Children* 1939, **58,** 102–118.

Rodbard, S. The clinical utility of the arterial pulses and sounds. *Heart and Lung* **1(6),** 776–784, November–December, 1972.

Rodbard, S., Rubinstein, H. M., and Rosenblum, S. Arrival time and calibrated contour of the pulse wave determined indirectly from re-

cordings of arterial compression sounds. *Am. Heart J.* 1957, **53,** 205–212.
Rodbard, S. and Mohrhers, R. Device for registration of the calibrated upstroke in man. *Rev. Sc. Instrs.* 1961, **32,** 1022–1023.
Rodbard, S. The clinical significance of the arterial sounds. *Heart Bull.* 1962, **11,** 41–45.
Rodbard, S. The significance of the intermittent Korotkoff sounds. *Circulation* 1953, **8,** 600–604.
Rodbard, S. In Segal, B. L. *Theory and Practice of Auscultation.* (Philadelphia: F. A. Davis Company, 1963), 562 pp.
Rodbard, S. and Lebanoff, A. J. Differentiation of aortic valve stenosis from subaortic muscular stenosis by means of arterial-sound recordings. *New England J. Med.* 1965, **273,** 780–784.
Rodbard, S. and Saiki, H. Flow through collapsible tubes. *Amer. Heart Journ.* 1953, **40,** 715–725.
Roman, J., Henry, J. P., and Meehan, J. P. Validity of flight blood pressure data. *Aerospace Med.* 1965, **36,** 436–446.
Segall, H. N. A note on the measurement of diastolic and systolic blood pressure by the palpation of arterial vibrations (sounds) over the brachial artery. *Canad. M.A.J.* 1940, **42,** 311–313.
Sewall H. Clinical significance of postural changes and the secondary waves of blood pressure. *Amer. Journ. Med Sci.* 1919, **158,** 786.
Siahaya, O., Kaku, A., and Ware, R. W. A digital readout technique applied to the laboratory and aerospace monitoring of physiological data. *S.A.M. Tech. Rep. TDR 62–139.* USAF Brooks AFB, TX, 1962.
Simpson, J. A., Jamieson, G., Dickhaus, D. W., and Grover, R. F. Effect of cuff bladder on accuracy of measurement of indirect blood pressure. *Amer. Heart Journ.* 1965, **70,** 208–215.
Steen, S. N. and Grissman, F. L. A new system for the indirect measurement of systolic and diastolic blood pressures. *Anesth. and Analg.* 1962, **41,** 391.
Stegall, H. F., Kardon, M. B., and Kemmerer, W. T. Indirect measurement of arterial blood pressure by Doppler ultrasonic sphygmomanometry. *J. Appl. Physiol.* 1968, **25,** 793–798.
Steinfeld, L., Alexander, H., and Cohen, M. L. Updating sphygmomanometry. *Amer. Journ. Cardiol.* 1974, **33,** 107–110.
Tavel, M., Faris, J., Nasser, W. K., Feigenbaum, H., and Fisch, C. Korotkoff sounds. *Circulation* 1969, **39,** 465–474.
Trout, K. W., Bertrand, C. A., and Williams, M. H. Measurement of blood pressure in obese persons. *Journ. Amer. Med. Assn.* 1956, **162,** 970-971.
Van Bergen, F. H., Weatherhead, D. S., Treolar, A. E., Dobkin, A. B., and Buckley, J. J. Comparison of indirect and direct methods of measuring arterial blood pressure. *Circulation* 1954, **10,** 481–490.
Von Recklinghausen, H. Über Blutdruckmessung beim Menschen. *Arch. Exper. Path. u. Pharmakol.* 1901, **46,** 78–132.
Wallace, J. D., Lewis, D. H., and Khalal, S. A. Korotkoff sound in human.

Journ. Accoust. Soc. Amer. 1961, **33,** 1178–1182.

Ware, R. W. and Kahn, A. R. Automatic indirect blood pressure determination in flight. J. Appl. Physiol. 1963, **18,** 210–214.

Ware, R. W. and Anderson, W. L. Spectral analysis of Korotkoff sounds. *IEEE Tr. on Biomed. Eng.* 1966, **BME–13,** 170–174.

Ware, R. W., Laenger, C. J., Heath, C. A., and Crosby, R. J. Development of indirect blood pressure sensing technique for aerospace vehicle and simulation use. *Tech. Rep. AMRL–TR–67–201.* Aerospace Res. Labs. Wright-Patterson AFB, Ohio, 1968, 137 pp.

Ware, R. W. and Laenger, C. J. Indirect blood pressure measurement by Doppler ultrasound kinetoarteriography. *Proc. 20th Ann. Conf. on Eng. in Med. and Biol.* (Boston) (Wellesley, Mass.: Wellesley Press, 1967).

Ware, R. W. and Laenger, C. J. Indirect recording of the entire arterial pressure wave. *Proc. 19th Ann. Conf. on Eng. in Med. and Biol.* 1966, **8,** 803. (San Francisco). Washington, 1966, McGregor and Werner.

Weaver, J. C. and Bohr, D. F. The digital blood pressure. *Amer. Heart Journ.* 1950, **39,** 413–422.

Wessale, J. L., Smith, L. A., Reed, M. E., Janas, W., Carter, A. B., and Geddes, L. A. Indirect auscultatory systolic and diastolic pressures in the anesthetized dog. *Amer. Journ. Vet. Res.* 1985, **46(10),** 2139–2132.

Whitcher, C. E. Department of Anesthesia, Stanford Medical Center, Palo Alto, California. Personal communication, 1962.

Whitcher, C. E., Cole, C. A., and Weaver, C. S. Stethoscope performance in transduction of human Korotkov blood pressure sounds (personal communication). *Presented to the Ann. Mtg. Am. Soc. Anesthesiologists,* 1967.

Whitcher, C. E., Smith, Ty, Cole, C. A., Manley, P. E., Weaver, C. S., Huntington, D. A., and Dixon, R. F. Analysis of human Korotkov sounds (personal communication). *Presented to the Ann. Mtg. Am. Soc. Anesthesiologists,* 1966.

Woodbury, R. A., Robinow, M., and Hamilton, W. F. Blood pressure studies on infants. *Amer. Journ. Physiol.* 1938, **122,** 472–479.

Wright, I. S., Schneider, R. F., and Ungerleider, H. E. Factors of error in blood pressure readings. *Am. Heart J.* 1938, **16,** 469–476.

Yamakoshi, K., Shimazu, H., and Togawa, T. Indirect measurement of instantaneous arterial blood pressure in the human finger by the vascular unloading technique. *IEEE Trans. Bio. Med. Eng.* 1980, **BME 27,** 150–155.

Yelderman, M. and Ream, A. K. Indirect measurement of mean blood pressure in the anesthetized patient. *Anesthesiol.* 1979, **50,** 253–256.

Yong, P. and Geddes, L. A. The effect of pressure deflation rate on accuracy in indirect measurement of blood pressure with the auscultatory method. *Journ. Clin. Mon.* 1987, **3(3),** 155–159.

Yong, P. and Geddes, L. A. A surrogate arm for evaluating the accuracy of indirect pressure-measuring instruments. *Biomed. Tech. Med. Instr.* 1990, **24(2),** 130–135.

PART THREE

History

INTRODUCTION

Instruments have played an essential role in quantifying blood pressure and allowing the conduct of experiments that identify the various factors that control it. Therefore, a short history of the evolution of these instruments is appropriate.

The concept of pressure was slow to evolve. Despite the extensive waterworks constructed by the Romans, they had no concept of pressure (force per unit area). "Water seeks its own level" was a satisfactory explanation for the agent that caused flow. The modern concept of pressure derives from an interest in the weight of the atmosphere, i.e., atmospheric pressure plus an interest in the compressibility of gases in the middle 1600s. Despite the clear definition of pressure at that time, the terms force and pressure were used interchangeably for some time.

EARLY OBSERVATIONS

Perhaps the best place to start the history of blood pressure is to identify its earliest manifestation, the pulse. With great ceremony and ritual, the ancient Chinese palpated the pulse bilaterally at 12 sites on the body surface, and believed that the nature of the pulse reflected the function of a specific organ. For example, the pulse at the right wrist identified the function of the lungs and large intestine. The left-wrist pulse reported on the function of the small intestine and heart. Other organs were studied by assessing the pulse at other sites.

Hippocrates (460–370 BC), the father of medicine, had no clear understanding of the meaning of the arterial pulse, despite his considerable contribution to codifying signs and symptoms with their prognostic implications. Without an accurate knowledge of the circulation, Galen (130–200 AD) was well aware of the cardiac origin of the pulse. He wrote a treatise on it in which he identified 27 varieties of the pulse. The true significance of the arterial pulse had to await discovery of the circulation in 1628 by William Harvey (1578–1657). By brilliant deduction, experiments on himself and animals, he proved that blood must move in a circle from the aorta to the veins and through the right heart to the lungs, thence to the left heart. His explanation and experiments appear in *De Motu Cordis*. However, he did not measure blood pressure.

The first to measure blood pressure was the Reverend Stephen Hales in 1733, in an unanesthetized horse (Fig. 1). In his book *Haemostaticks*, he wrote:

> "1. In December I caused a Mare to be tied down alive on her Back, she was fourteen Hands high, and about fourteen Years of Age, had a Fistula on her Withers, was neither very lean, nor yet lusty: Having laid open the crural Artery about three Inches from her Belly, I inserted into it a brass Pipe whose Bore was one sixth of an Inch in Diameter; and to that, by means of another brass Pipe which was fitly adapted to it, I fixed a glass Tube, of nearly the same Diameter, which was nine Feet in Length. Then untying the Ligature on the Artery, the Blood rose in the Tube eight Feet three Inches perpendicular above the Level of the left Ventricle of the Heart: But it did not attain to its full Height at once; it rushed up about half way in an Instant, and afterwards gradually at each Pulse twelve, eight, six, four, two, and sometimes one Inch: When it was at its full Height, it would rise and fall at and after each Pulse two, three, or four Inches; and sometimes it would fall twelve or fourteen Inches, and have there for a time the same Vibrations up and down at and after each Pulse, as it had, when it was at its full Height; to which it would rise again, after forty or fifty Pulses.
>
> The Pulse of a Horse that is well, and not terrified, nor in any Pain, is about thirty six Beats in a Minute, which is nearly half as fast as the Pulse of a Man in Health: This Mare's Pulse beat about fifty five times in a Minute, and sometimes sixty or a hundred she being in pain."

Hales wrote in old English that capitalizes the nouns, as in German. He used terms that are less familiar today. For example, fourteen hands equals 56 inches. A fistula on her withers describes an erosive skin lesion over the shoulders, probably caused by a harness. The crural artery is the femoral artery. The pressure equivalent to 8-feet-three inches in mm Hg is $8 \times 12'' + 3'' = 99$ inch of blood. Assuming a density of 1 gm/mL for blood, and 13.56 for

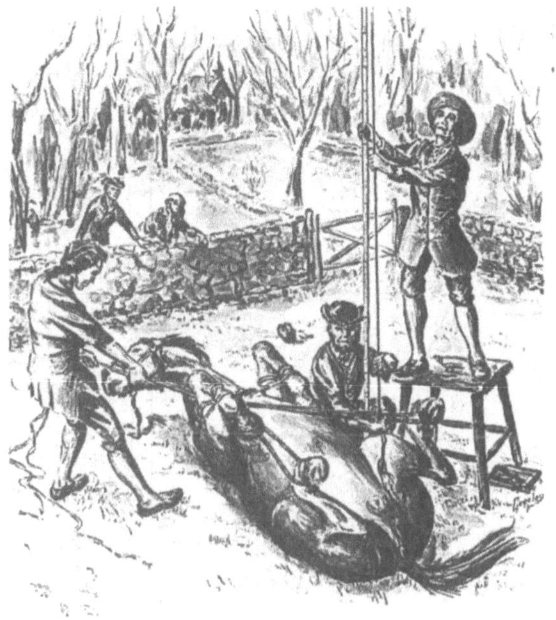

Fig. 1. Artist's concept drawn from Hales' account of the first direct measurement of arterial pressure in 1733.

mercury, the equivalent pressure is (99 × 25.4)/13.56 = 185.4 mm Hg. Although this pressure is high for the horse, it should be remembered that the animal was not anesthetized. It is clear that Hales saw both the pulsatile cardiac and respiratory variations (12–14 inches) in blood pressure.

It is less well known that Hales was the first to study hemorrhagic shock. Again using the horse, he withdrew blood and measured the pressure after withdrawing each quart. Figure 2 is a summary of his results. Observe that the blood pressure fell progressively until about eight quarts of blood were removed, at which point the blood pressure stabilized until about 13 quarts were removed, following which compensation was no longer possible.

Obviously, it was impractical to use a tall vertical tube to measure arterial pressure. A solution to this problem was introduced by Poiseuille (1828), who employed the mercury-filled, U tube manometer. By using mercury, the height supported by pressure was reduced 13.56-fold. By using the U tube with equal arms, the height that the mercury rose in one arm of the U tube was reduced by a factor of two (*see* Part 1). Poiseuille's manometer is shown in Fig. 1, Part 1. Not only did Poiseuille make the measure-

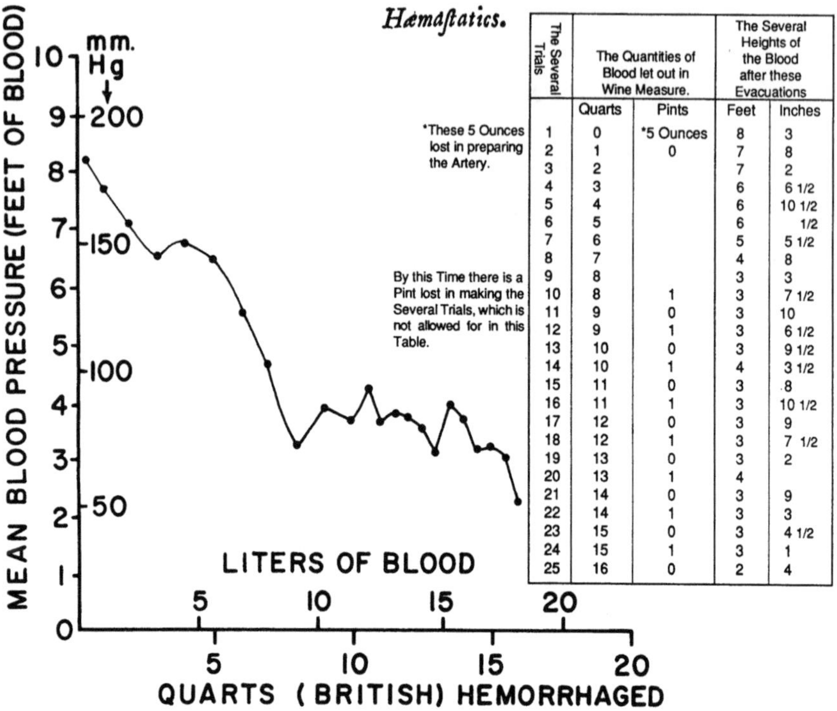

The Several Trials	The Quantities of Blood let out in Wine Measure.		The Several Heights of the Blood after these Evacuations	
	Quarts	Pints	Feet	Inches
1	0	*5 Ounces	8	3
2	1	0	7	8
3	2		7	2
4	3		6	6 1/2
5	4		6	10 1/2
6	5		6	1/2
7	6		5	5 1/2
8	7		4	8
9	8		3	3
10	8	1	3	7 1/2
11	9	0	3	10
12	9	1	3	6 1/2
13	10	0	3	9 1/2
14	10	1	4	3 1/2
15	11	0	3	.8
16	11	1	3	10 1/2
17	12	0	3	9
18	12	1	3	7 1/2
19	13	0	3	2
20	13	1	4	
21	14	0	3	9
22	14	1	3	3
23	15	0	3	4 1/2
24	15	1	3	1
25	16	0	2	4

*These 5 Ounces lost in preparing the Artery.

By this Time there is a Pint lost in making the Several Trials, which is not allowed for in this Table.

Fig. 2. The first study of hemorrhagic shock carried out by Hales. Shown here is blood pressure vs the vol of blood removed from a horse. Hales' original data appear in the inset. (From Hales, S., *Haemastaticks,* 1738.)

ment of blood pressure practical, he gave us our units for blood pressure, mm Hg. Interestingly, the title of his thesis, for which he was awarded the MD degree, is "The Force of the Aortic Heart."

The mercury U-tube manometer could be duplicated easily, and investigators began to use it to measure blood pressure. However, the U-tube manometer was known long before Poiseuille. In Fact, Hales used one to measure the pressure of sap in plants; Fig. 3 is an illustration of Hales' sap manometer.

DIRECT RECORDERS

Measuring the height of the mercury column in the U-tube was difficult. A solution to this problem was presented by Ludwig (1847), who introduced graphic recording to physiology and medicine. However, graphic recording had been in use for some time in meterology by Ons-en-Bray (1734) (*see* Hoff and Geddes, 1957).

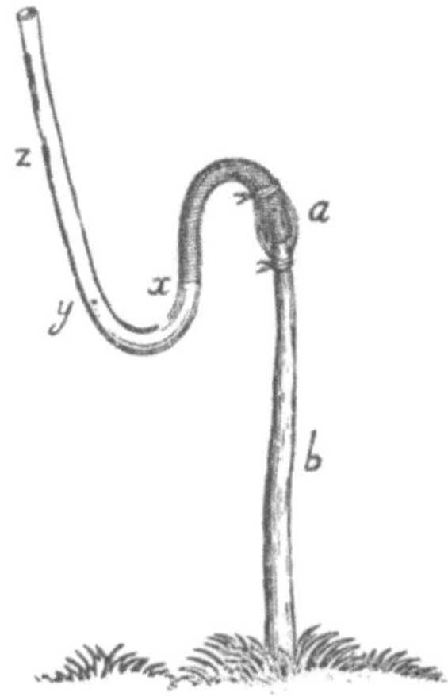

Fig. 3. Hales' U-tube manometer, to measure the pressure of sap in plants. (From Hales, S., *Vegetable Stabicks,* 1738.)

This, however, in no way diminishes Ludwig's contribution. It was the introduction of the smoked-drum kymograph (wave recorder) that ushered in the scientific era of blood-pressure measurement.

Figure 4A illustrates Ludwig's smoked-drum kymograph that was first driven by a falling weight (w). A float on the mercury in the open tube supported a slender rod (cc) to which a stylus (gf) was affixed. The tip of the stylus scratched soot from the rotating smoked drum, thereby displaying a graphic record of blood pressure. Figure 4B is Ludwig's recording of carotid artery pressure in a morphinized dog. Observe the large-amplitude variations owing to the slow deep breathing, and the sinus arrhythmia, both characteristic of the morphinized animal.

Although the small-amplitude cardiac oscillations are clearly evident in Fig. 4B, it was appreciated that their true amplitude was not accurately displayed, owing to the considerable inertia of the mercury column and the appreciable fluid friction. Therefore, the pressure displayed by the mercury manometer was mean pressure with superimposed cardiac and respiratory variations. There soon ensued a race to create instruments that would display blood pressure faithfully. Fick (1864) was the first to devise a rapidly responding, direct-writing instrument that consisted of a tube that was flattened slightly and bent into the shape of a C, as shown in Fig. 5A. Because the outer area of the C is slightly larger than the inner, the application of pressure via the lead tube (r) caused the C to uncurl slightly. To the free end of the tube was affixed a linkage (h)

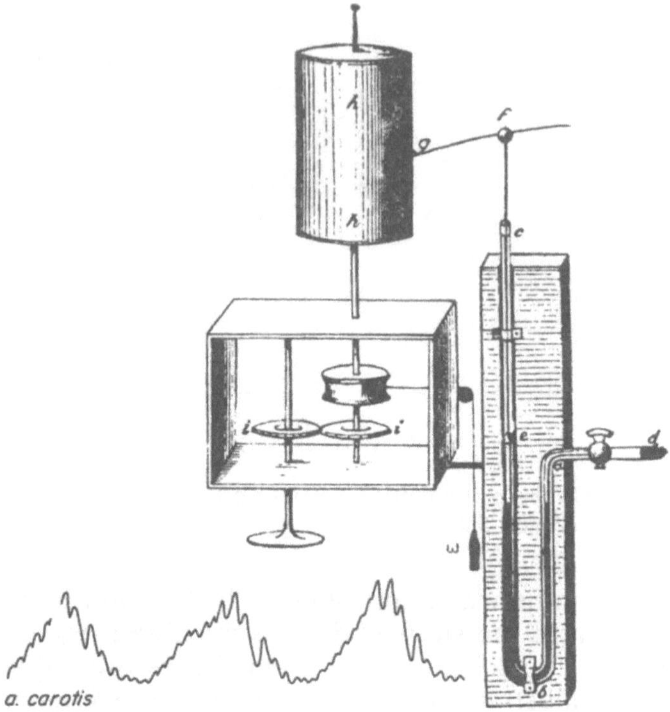

Fig. 4. Ludwig's smoked-drum kymograph (hh) and mercury manometer with a float (cc) supporting a writing stylus (g). (From Ludwig, C., 1847.)

that was coupled to a second linkage (h′) that in turn was coupled to two other arms (h″ h‴). To h″ was affixed a stylus (S) and a small disk (P) that was placed in a fluid to provide viscous damping to prevent the system from overshooting when a rapid change in pressure occurred. Figure 5B shows a record made with Fick's C-spring recorder. Just past the center of the record, the heart rate was reduced (probably by vagal stimulation). Note the absence of a dicrotic notch, indicating that the response time was long.

The outstanding difference between the records obtained with the mercury manometer (Fig. 4B) and the C-spring recorder (Fig. 5B) was the amplitude of the pulsations. How large they should be was unknown, and renewed efforts were made to shorten the response time. Fick (1883) introduced his straight-spring recorder that is shown in Fig. 6A. It consisted of a small chamber (b) covered by a diaphragm (c) having a projection (d) that pressed against a leaf spring (f) that was coupled to a long member (g) that drove the pivoted writing lever (h). Figure 6B is a record of aortic and left-

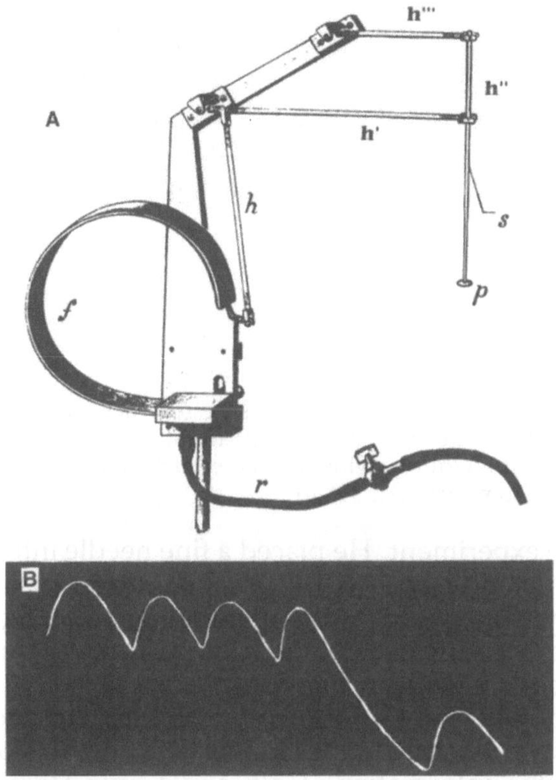

Fig. 5. Fick's C-spring blood-pressure recorder. Pressure applied to the fluid-filled lead tube (r) caused the C spring to uncurl slightly. To the tip of the C was affixed a train of levers carrying the stylus (S) that scratched soot from a smoked-drum kymograph (From Fick, A., 1864.)

ventricular pressure (not recorded simultaneously). Observe the slight hint of a dicrotic notch on the aortic pressure waveform, and the small-amplitude oscillations near left-ventricular systolic pressure.

During this time, many different instruments were used for recording blood pressure directly. The records obtained were often quite different. Some thought that the small-amplitude oscillations seen in many records were genuine events; others believed that they were produced by the instruments, and had no physiological basis. Particularly controversial was the dicrotic notch, reproduction of which required a rapidly responding recorder.

With only a kymograph and no mechanical recorder, Landois (1874) demonstrated the presence of the dicrotic notch by an ele-

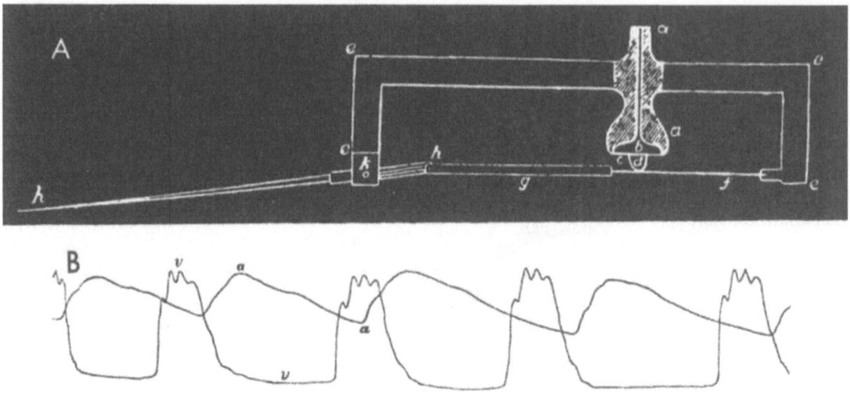

Fig. 6. Fick's straight-spring blood pressure recorder (A). Pressure applied to the diaphragm (c) caused the leaf spring (f) to move downward, resulting in an upward motion of the writing stylus (h) that scratched soot from a smoked-drum kymograph (B). (From Fick, A., 1883.)

gantly simple experiment. He placed a fine needle into an artery and directed the jet of blood to the rotating drum of a kymograph. There, clearly displayed was the dicrotic notch, along with systolic and diastolic pressures. He called his record a hemautograph, a copy of which is shown in Fig. 7.

Not only was there doubt about the dicrotic notch, there was controversy over the true values for systolic and diastolic pressures. To provide this information, Golz and Gaule (1878) equipped a mercury manometer with two oppositely directed check valves and a selector valve that could connect the manometer to the artery via one check valve or the other. The technique they used is sketched in Fig. 8. With the system fluid-filled, the selector valve was placed in position "Systolic," that connected the manometer to the artery so that, with each heart beat, blood would flow from the artery through the upper check valve into the manometer. Because the valve permitted only forward flow, when arterial pressure started to fall, the fluid in the manometer would force the check valve shut. After a few heart beats, the height of the manometer displayed the maximum systolic pressure attained during the period of recording. To measure diastolic pressure, the selector valve was turned clockwise one quarter turn to the "Diastolic" position, and the fluid in the manometer forced the lower check valve open when arterial pressure was below the pressure in the manometer. After a few beats, the reading on the mercury manometer fell to the minimum diastolic pressure occurring during the period of recording. Thus, with this simple device coupled to the slowly responding mercury

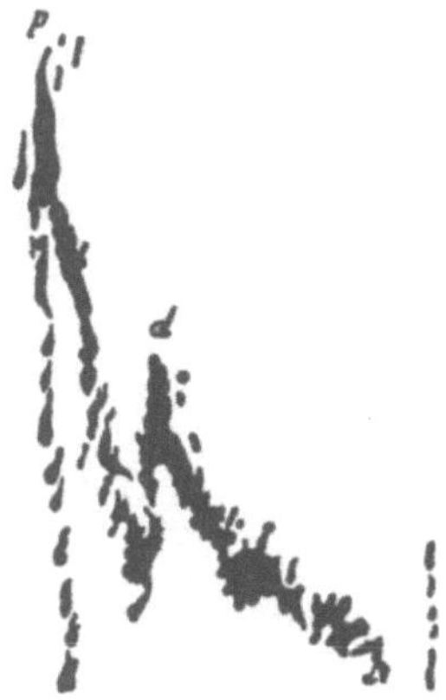

Fig. 7. Landois' hemantogram, a record of blood pressure made by directing a fine jet of arterial blood against a moving chart. Clearly displayed is the dicrotic notch. (From Luciani, L., *Human Physiology*, trans. by F. A. Welby, Macmillan & Co., Ltd., London, 1911, **9**, 71, vol. 1, 592 pp.)

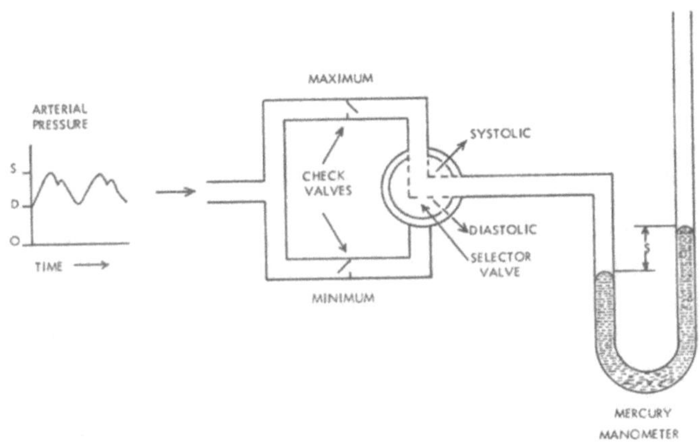

Fig. 8. The maximum and minimum pressure manometer used by Golz and Gaule to determine systolic and diastolic pressures with the mercury manometer.

manometer, systolic and diastolic pressures could be measured with accuracy.

A different approach to the measurement of blood pressure was taken by Marey (1881), who became the champion of the graphic method for a remarkable variety of physiological events, as well as the gaits of runners and horses, and the flight of birds. Whereas all previous investigators used fluid-filled systems with considerable inertia and fluid friction, Marey perfected the air-filled system for recording blood pressure shown in Fig. 9. Pressure was detected by a special sound (OV), consisting of a small cage mounted to the end

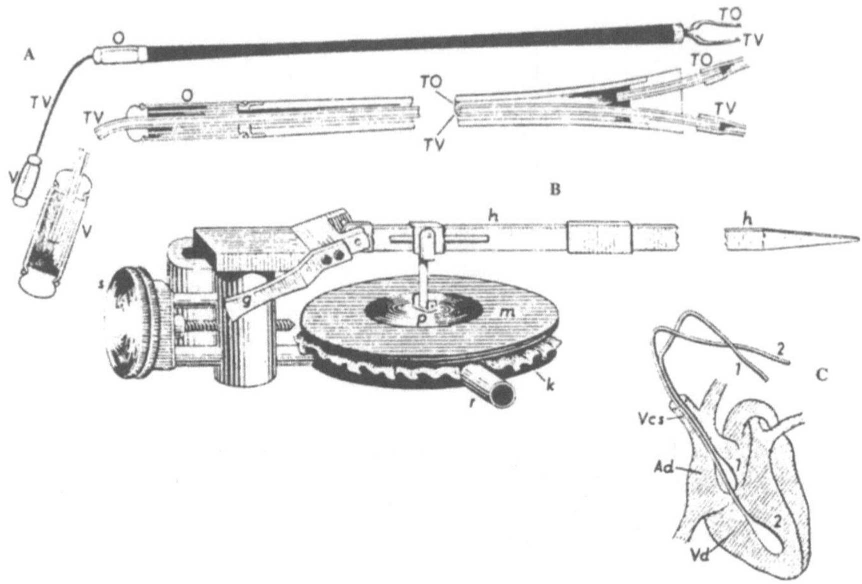

Fig. 9. Marey's pneumatic system for measuring blood pressure. A illustrates a double O (atrial) and V (ventricle) sound. In B is shown the recording tambour, the stylus (h) of which scratched soot from a smoked-drum kymograph. In C is shown the location of the sounds in the right atrium (Ad), and right ventricle (Vd). (Redrawn from Marey, E. J., *La Circulation du Sang*, G. Mason, Paris, 1881, 745 pp.)

of a metal catheter. The cage was covered with a rubber membrane; the space inside was connected to a tambour (m). When pressure was applied to the sound, the rubber on the sound was pressed inward, and the pressure change was recorded by the tambour writing lever (h). With this equipment, Marey recorded aortic pressure, left and right ventricular pressures, and right atrial pressure in the unanesthetized horse. One of his remarkable recordings, the first accurate catheter records of cardiac chamber pressure, is shown in Fig. 10. Calibration was achieved by placing the sounds at different depths in water. When calibrated, these records clearly showed that, ventricular pressure fell to near zero during diastole. They also showed the rapid rise and fall of ventricular pressure, and the time in the cardiac cycle when the aortic valve opened and closed.

The beginning of the end of the era of direct recorders began in 1888 when Hurthle improved Fick's straight spring recorder by increasing the stiffness of the leaf spring and using a short, lightweight writing lever; Fig. 11 illustrates Hurthle's instrument and a recording obtained with it. Depending on the design, the natural resonant frequency was between 10 and 20 Hz. An amplitude of 10–

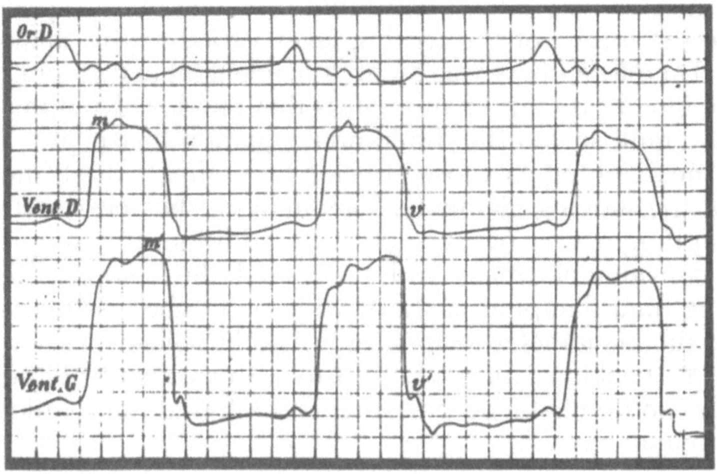

Fig. 10. Right-atrial (OrD), right ventricular (Vent. D), and left ventricular (Vent. G) pressures recovered by Marey, using the pneumatic system shown in Fig. 10.

A

S

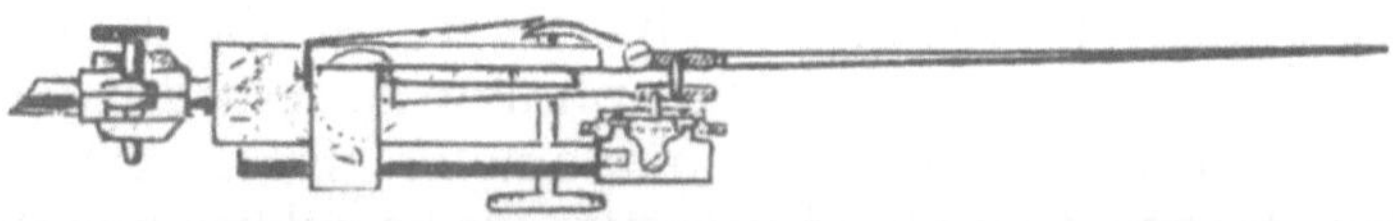

B

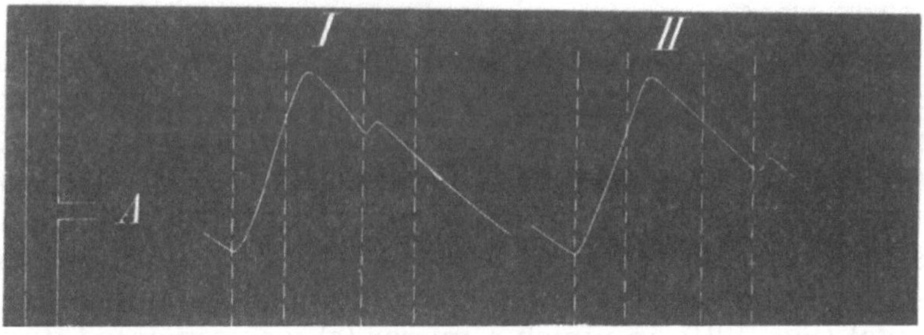

Fig. 11. The last direct-writing blood pressure manometer introduced by Hurthle in 1888 (A). The maximum recording amplitude was 20 mm for 100 mm Hg. The tip of the writing lever (S) scratched soot from a rotating smoked-drum kymograph. In B is shown one of Hurthle's records of blood pressure, revealing the dicrotic notch. (Redrawn from Hurthle, 1890.)

20 mm on the record represented 100 mm Hg. Use of this instrument persisted well into the 20th century.

By the late 1800s, it was becoming obvious that the moving mass had to be small, and that the diaphragm that was deflected by blood pressure had to be stiff. However, the consequence of using a stiff diaphragm was a loss of sensitivity. Adding a long writing lever to regain sensitivity added mass that prolonged the response time because the inertia of the writing lever varied as the square of its length. Therefore, there was an undeniable limit to further improvement of blood pressure manometers that employed writing levers. In 1903, Frank solved the differential equation that relates the motion of the diaphragm exposed to blood pressure to its stiffness, and mass of the moving elements. The analysis showed clearly that a stiff diaphragm was needed, and the addition of a writing lever added considerable mass and prolonged the response time. To minimize fluid damping, a short, wide-bore tube was necessary to connect the manometer to an artery. Another means was obviously needed to enable display of the tiny displacement of the elastic member exposed to blood pressure; Frank found the solution in the optical manometer.

OPTICAL MANOMETERS

In 1924, Frank described his "light" lever, i.e., the use of a beam of light reflected from the elastic diaphragm to record blood pressure photographically. In Frank's manometer (Fig. 12A), the elastic member deflected by blood pressure was a rubber membrane stiffened by a leaf spring that carried the mirror. From the data presented by Frank, the natural frequency was 300 Hz, and the vol displacement was calculated to be about 1 cu mm/100 mm Hg. Although Frank used this device for many years, he did not describe it until 1924. During this time, Wiggers (1914, 1924) also stressed the need for a high natural frequency for the faithful reproduction of the pressure transients existing in the vascular system. To measure these, he described his own version of Frank's manometer (segment capsule) (Fig. 12B), in which a mirror (c) was cemented directly to the stiff rubber membrane, thereby eliminating the leaf spring Frank had used. In Wiggers' instrument, the light beam reflected from the mirror on the membrane was first reflected from a stationary mirror mounted above it. A second light beam reflected from this stationary mirror to the screen provided a zero pressure baseline on the photographic record. Desirous of obtaining an even shorter response time and smaller vol displacement than that available with Wiggers' manometer, Hamilton (1934) constructed his own optical manometer that employed a brass membrane 60-μ thick, and about 5 mm in diameter (Fig. 12C). A mirror (M) was mounted on a thin triangular rubber cushion that, in turn, was cemented to the brass

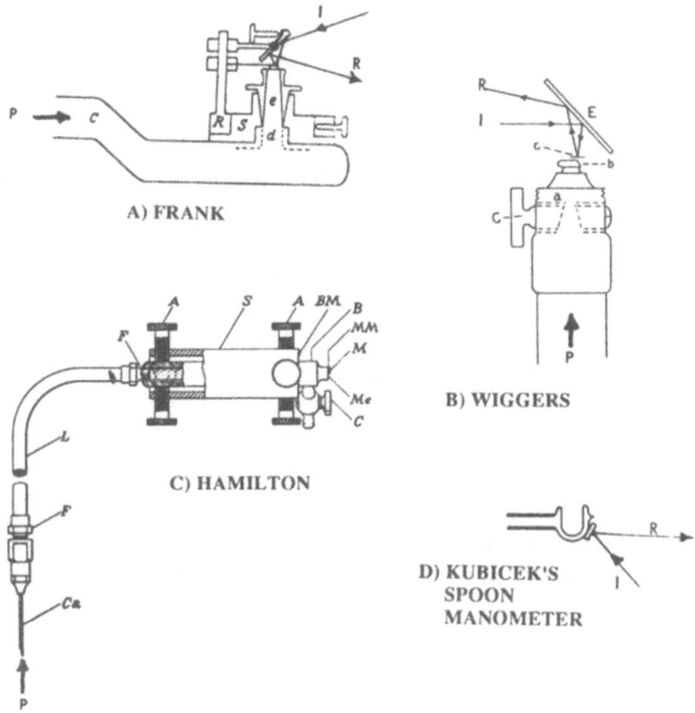

Fig. 12. The optical manometers. I = incident beam; R = reflected beam. A, Frank (Redrawn from Frank, O., *Zschr. Biol.* **82,** 49–65, 1924). B, Wiggers (Redrawn from Wiggers, C. J., *Am. J. Physiol.* **33,** 382–396, 1914). C, Hamilton (Redrawn from Hamilton, W. F., et al., *Am. J. Physiol.* **107,** 427–435, 1934). D, Kubicek's spoon manometer (Redrawn from *Medical Physics*, vol. 1, Year Book Medical Publishers, Inc., Chicago, 1944).

membrane (ME). Because of the increased stiffness provided by the brass membrane, adequate sensitivity was obtained by increasing the distance from the mirror on the membrane to the recording photographic surface to about 5 to 6 meters.

The Hamilton manometer became the standard in the US until well after the end of World War II (1945). Its performance characteristics were excellent. Using lead tubing (10–20 cm × 0.5 mm) and small-bore needles (16–20 ga), resonant frequencies of 200–250 Hz were routinely attained when great care was taken to exclude all air bubbles. The vol displacement of the best model was on the order of 0.02 cu mm/100 mm Hg.

The use of shim brass for the membrane deflected by blood pressure encountered difficulties, e.g., maintenance of a fluid-tight seal for the diaphragm and metal fatigue after prolonged use. To solve these problems, glass membranes were used. Broemser (1927) installed one into a Frank-type manometer to obtain a natural frequency of 250 Hz. Kubicek et al. (1941) developed a one-piece glass spoon manometer that was made by first blowing a bubble (10 mm diam) on the end of a 2.5 mm glass tube; it was then heated over part of its surface by a pointed flame to form the spoon. A small concave mirror was mounted on the tip of the spoon (Fig. 12D); photographic recording was used.

Optical manometers provided high-fidelity recordings of blood pressure waves wherever they were measured in the vascular system, and much fundamental knowledge was gained through their use. However, optical manometers presented practical difficulties. For example, to obtain adequate sensitivity, the photographic recording surface had to be placed from five to fifteen feet from the manometer. Stray light entering the recording surface caused difficulties and, because of the long optical pathway, all the apparatus had to be rigidly mounted to avoid recording vibrations caused by activities in the building, and seismic vibrations. Most inconvenient was the need to locate the subject very close to the fixed-site manometer with lead tubing. Finally, it was necessary to wait for developing, and fixing the photographic record before viewing it. Despite these inconveniences, the optical manometers survived until the mid 1950s.

ELECTRICAL MANOMETERS

Catheter Type

Whereas the direct-writing blood-pressure records were undergoing their final stages of perfection, the first electrically operated blood-pressure manometer was developed by Grunbaum (1898). What is even more remarkable is that it was a catheter-tip unit, a description of which appears in the section in this chapter that deals with the history of catheter-tip transducers.

All electrically operated blood-pressure transducers employ the electrical detection of the deflection of an elastic member exposed to blood pressure. Many different methods (resistive, capacitive, inductive, and photoelectric) have been used to derive an electrical signal from deflection of the elastic member. The major advantage of the electrical manometers lies in the fact that a long cable can be used for connection to the display device, without a loss of fidelity. Even before De Forest's (1906) introduction of the vacuum tube with its amplifying capabilities, there were sensitive, rapidly responding graphic recorders, such as Thompson's reflecting galvanometer (1850) (*see* Geddes, 1987), the Lippmann capillary electrometer (*see* Geddes and Hoff, 1961), the Siemen-Halske and Dudell oscillographs (for recording alternating current waveforms), as well as the Einthoven string galvanometer (1903). Therefore, all that was needed was skillful application of electrical methods to detect the tiny displacement of the elastic member exposed to blood pressure.

As stated previously, the first electrical blood pressure transducer was a catheter-tip unit. It is described along with the other catheter-tip units. The principle it employed was used in many of the first pressure transducers.

In 1916 Garten constructed a manometer in which the rubber membrane was stiff, and pressure applied to it altered the cross-sectional area of an electrolyte between the electrodes. Figure 13A is a sketch of this device, that consisted of a T-shaped glass container with two electrodes (Z_1, Z_2), and filled with zinc sulfate solution. A partition (D) divided the container almost in half. On one side of the device was placed a stiff rubber membrane (G), that was exposed to the pressure to be measured. Below the membrane was a mound of paraffin wax, arranged so that only a thin column of electrolyte provided a conduction path between Z_1 and Z_2. When pressure was applied to G, via the coupling unit (H), the cross-sectional area of the thin column of electrolyte was reduced, thereby increasing the resistance. A string galvanometer was used to record the pressure.

The first to introduce what could be called a modern transducer was Schutz (1937), who constructed a capacitive manometer in which the elastic member was a silvered glass plate that exhibited a resonant frequency of 270 Hz when exposed to a step function of pressure. Although Schutz presented few additional details, he reported that his device was entirely satisfactory for recording blood pressure anywhere in the circulatory system, and that his oscillator-amplifier-oscillograph recording system provided records of large amplitude.

Rein (1940) used the photoelectric method to detect the motion of the tip of Fick's C-spring (Bourdon tube) manometer. Rein's instrument, illustrated in Fig. 13B employed a hinged vane (Bb), coupled to the free end of the Bourdon tube (MF). Opposite the hinged vane was another vane (Bf) that was adjustable to close the intervening space. Below the two vanes was a photocell, and above

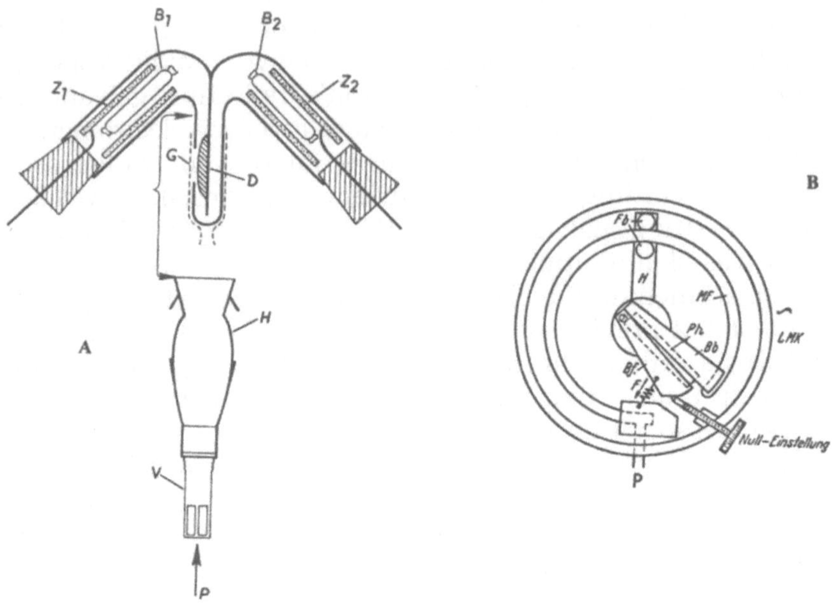

Fig. 13. The first electrical catheter-type blood-pressure transducers (A, Garten, 1916; B, Rein, 1940).

was placed a one-third watt exciter lamp. Pressure applied to the Bourdon tube caused the space between the two vanes to enlarge and expose the photocell to the exciter lamp. The output of the photocell energized a recording oscillograph; no amplification was used.

The performance characteristics of Rein's photoelectric transducer were such that, it could be used confidently with a cannula 12 cm in length, and 4 mm in diameter. The transducer-recorder system was linear, and provided a maximum sensitivity of 1200 mm/mm Hg. The fluid-filled resonant frequency was 44 Hz, with a damping factor of 0.6–0.8. The vol displacement was quite high, being 13.5 cu mm/100 mm Hg; a figure, that, as Rein stated, requires the use of large-bore catheters or needles for faithful reproduction of the arterial pressure curve.

Probably because the Wiggers' manometer had gained such popularity but had the practical inconveniences of all optical manometers, Gilson (1943) adapted the photoelectric principle of transduction to it. In one application, as the pressure was applied, the light beam reflected from the mirror on the elastic membrane varied the amount of light reaching a photocathode. In another version,

Gilson mounted a shade on the elastic membrane and placed a light source on one side and a photodetector on the other. Pressure applied to the manometer caused the shade to alter the amount of light reaching the photocathode, thereby producing an electrical signal.

In 1876, Tomlinson reported that a wire, when strained, increases its resistance. Strain is defined as the increase in length, divided by the original length. Practical use of this phenomenon did not occur until 66 yr later, when Simmonds (1942) patented the phenomenon, and wires of carefully controlled composition (strain gauges) became available commercially. In physiology, the first practical use of strain gauges was described by Grundfest and Hay (1945), who constructed a sensitive pressure transducer that employed two strain gauges coupled to a diaphragm, exposed to the tiny pulsatile air-pressure changes occurring in a small chamber surrounding the first finger of a human subject. Although they did not report use of their strain-gauge transducer for the measurement of blood pressure, they proposed its use for this purpose. In the mid 1940s, Statham developed his well-known strain-gauge transducer (*see* Part 1), that made it easy to record blood pressure. The characteristics of this device were reported by Lambert and Wood (1947). They stated that its performance compared favorably with the standard at that time, the Hamilton optical manometer!

Catheter-Tip Transducers

The first catheter-tip transducer was also the first electrical transducer for blood pressure. In 1898, Grunbaum described his sound (transducer) for measuring pressure in the cardiac ventricles. Without the usual justification for devising his instrument, Grunbaum merely stated "The method consists of causing alteration of pressure to change the electric resistance of a circuit which thereby produces an alteration in the potential difference of two points which is recorded by photographing the meniscus of a capillary electrometer." Figure 14 is a diagram of the equipment used by Grunbaum. His instrument consisted of a capsule 3 mm in diameter (9F), and an ebonite cylinder affixed to the tip of a catheter. On one side of the capsule was a window covered with an elastic membrane that was deflected by the application of pressure (P). On the inner side of the membrane was mounted an amalgamated zinc electrode. Opposite it, and inside the capsule was fixed a similar zinc elec-

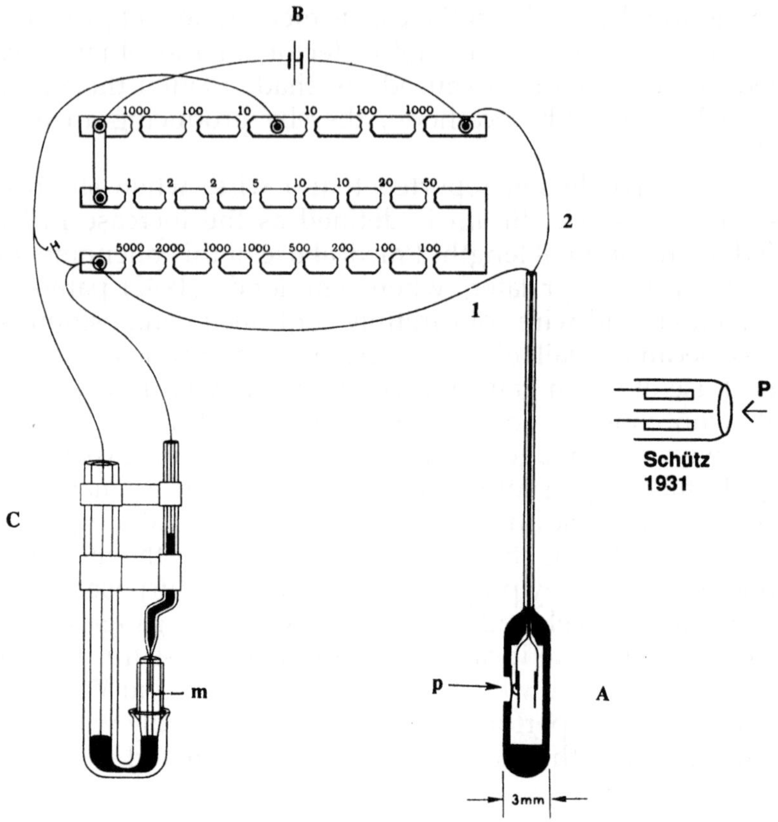

Fig. 14. Grunbaum's catheter-tip pressure transducer (A), a Wheatstone bridge (B), and the capillary electrometer (C). The resistance change owing to the applied pressure (P) altered the current through the mercury-sulfuric acid meniscus (m). A photographic recording of the change in the meniscus provided the pressure record. (Redrawn from Grunbaum, O. F. T., *Journ. Physiol.* 1897, 1898, **22,** XLIX-LI.)

trode. Between these two electrodes was an electrolyte (zinc sulfate). The electrodes were connected to insulated wires (1,2) that were brought out the end of the catheter. With an increase in pressure (P), the interelectrode distance decreased, thereby decreasing the resistance appearing between the two electrode wires (1,2). The electrodes were connected to a Wheatstone bridge (B), the output of which was connected to a capillary electrometer (C) (*see* Geddes and Hoff, 1961). The contour of the meniscus (m) of the capillary electrometer changed with the resistance change produced by the pressure applied to the catheter. A photographic recording of the contour of the mercury meniscus constituted a record of blood pressure. Grunbaum reported successful use of his catheter-tip pressure transducer in the right ventricle of a rabbit. However, his pressure recording has not been found.

The next catheter-tip transducer was also electrolytic. Whereas Grunbaum's unit was side-viewing (Fig. 14A) for pressure, the model built by Schutz (1931) was end-viewing for pressure. His instrument, shown in Fig. 15A, consisted of a glass tube, 5 mm diam., divided down the middle by an insulating partition that extended to within 0.3 mm of the end, over which was pulled a taut rubber membrane. In each compartment was a copper electrode, and the tube was then filled with copper sulfate. Pressure applied to the membrane decreased the area of the electrolytic conductor between the two electrodes, and hence increased the resistance of the device. Schutz used a string galvanometer to record pressure.

The performance characteristics of Schutz's device were excellent. It was linear with pressure between 20 and 200 mm Hg, and exhibited a natural frequency in air of 600–700 Hz, and in fluid about 200 Hz. Hence, the response time was remarkably short; in fact, it was so short that in his recordings of the right atrial pressure in the dog, there are clear vibrations that represent the first and second heart sounds.

Wagner (1932) improved Schutz's design and used a celluloid tube and partition, thereby adding practicality to the construction. Figure 15B illustrates the instrument that had a linear range of −130 + 50 mm Hg. The response time was probably limited by the string galvanometer that he used as a recorder. The transient response record published shows virtually no overshoot. With this recording system, Wagner presented records, showing the relationship between the variations in right ventricular pressure in the dog to the inspiratory and expiratory phases of respiration.

Although the electrolytic, catheter-tip strain gauge transducers had excellent dynamic response characteristics, were easy to make, and provided a relatively large resistance change per mm Hg, their lifetime was short, owing to electrochemical corrosion. Moreover, the temperature stability left something to be desired; typical electrolytes have a resistivity temperature coefficient of −2% per degree Centigrade. These two latter features resulted in abandonment of electrolytic pressure transducers.

Wetterer (1943) described a catheter-tip transducer that employed a differential transformer to detect the deflection of the elastic member exposed to blood pressure. His instrument, shown in Fig. 15C, consisted of a miniature four-winding differential transformer mounted inside the tip of a catheter 3.5 mm in diameter.

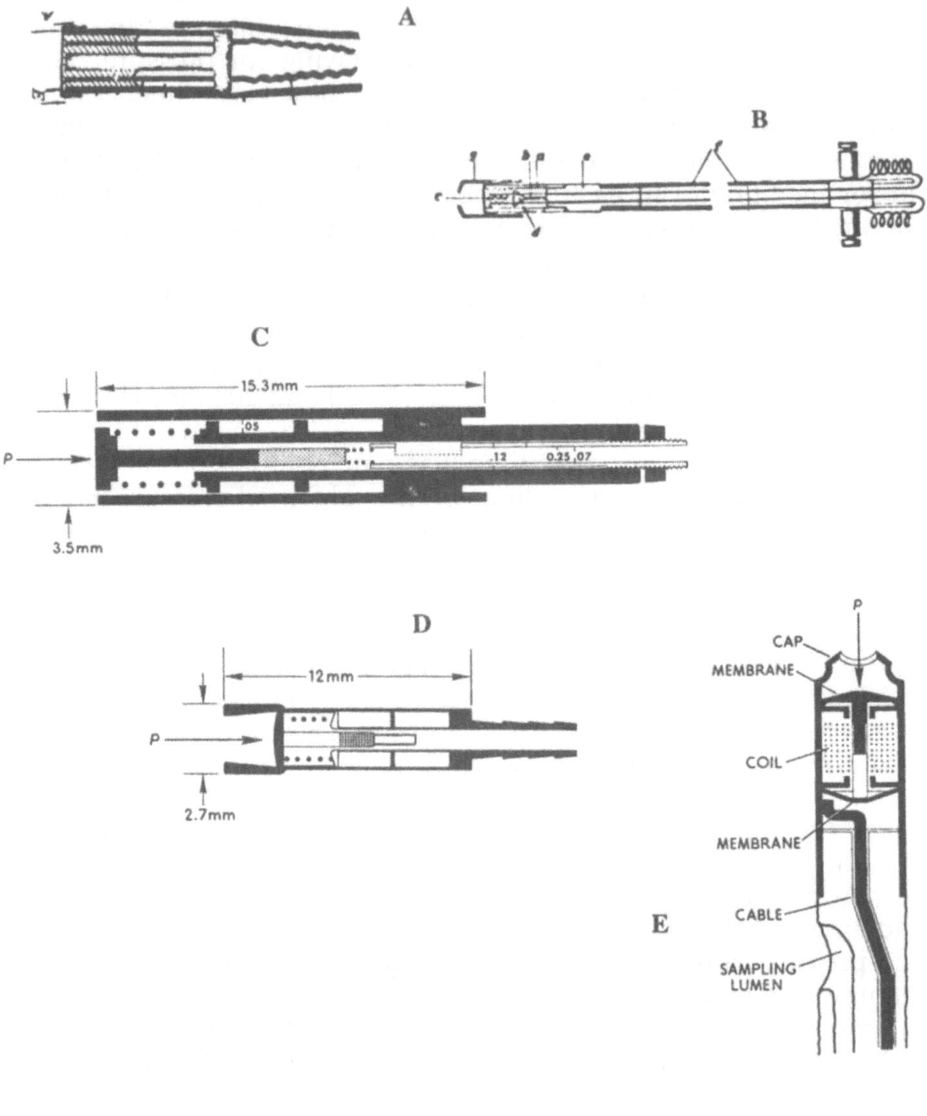

Fig. 15. Catheter-tip pressure transducers. A, Schutz electrolytic (Schutz, E., *Zeits, Biol.* 1931, **91,** 515–521); B, Wagner's electrolytic (*Zeits, Biol.* 1932, **92,** 54–85); C, Wetterer's differential transformer (*Zeits, Biol.* 1943, **101,** 332–350); D, Gauer and Gienapp, differential transformer (*Science* 1950, **112,** 404–405); and E, Laurens' variable inductance (*Arch. Mal de Coeur* 1959, **52,** 121–132). All illustrations redrawn from references cited.

Two of the windings were connected in series-aiding, and constituted the primary coil to which a 6000-Hz oscillator was connected. The other two windings were wired in series-opposition, and connected to the measuring apparatus. The symmetrically placed core of the transformer was coupled to a spring that pressed it against a rubber membrane mounted on the end of the catheter. Pressure applied to the membrane altered the position of the core and unbalanced the symmetry of the voltages induced in the windings connected in series-opposition, causing the appearance of a 6000-Hz voltage that was processed for display. With this equipment, Wetterer presented recordings of intrathoracic and the pressure in the right jugular vein of the rabbit.

The performance characteristics of Wetterer's catheter-tip transducer were very good. The diaphragm was light, and the stiffness was high, resulting in a natural frequency of 515 Hz. It was linear, and with a two-stage amplifier and a recording oscillograph, Wetterer reported a sensitivity of 20 mm/mm Hg.

By the end of the 1940s, there was an increased interest in using catheter-tip transducers to eliminate the long, fluid-filled catheter that limited the ability of a transducer to respond rapidly. In the US, Gauer and Gienapp (1950) devised a catheter-tip transducer similar to that described by Wetterer (1943); the Gauer-Gienapp transducer is shown in Fig. 15D. The core of a differential transformer was affixed to a stiff membrane mounted to the end of an 8F catheter. The device had a resonant frequency of 1000 Hz in fluid, with a damping factor of 0.34. A notable feature of this transducer was the addition of a 2-mm long open cylinder at the end of the catheter. This accessory minimized movement artifacts by preventing the diaphragm from striking vessel or cavity walls. An excellent pullback record of left ventricular and aortic pressure in the dog appears in their paper.

None of the catheter-tip transducers just described were available commercially; although the Gauer-Gienapp unit was duplicated for a few investigators. Laurens (1959) described a variable-inductance, catheter-tip transducer that became available commercially (Telco Inc., Paris and Dallons-Telco, Los Angeles, CA). The Laurens transducer was originally described at the 1954 Second World Congress of Cardiology. Figure 15E illustrates the transducer mounted at the tip of a two-lumen 8F catheter; it also incorporated a protective cap to minimize flailing artifacts. One lumen of the catheter was used for the two wires from the transducer; the other was open to permit withdrawal of a blood sample or injection of a radiopaque substance at the site of pressure measurement. Pressure applied to the membrane at the end of the catheter advanced a Mumetal core farther into a single coil, thereby increasing its inductance. The inductance formed part of the frequency-determining circuit of an oscillator. The increase in inductance lowered the frequency of the oscillator, thereby creating a frequency modulation system. The electronic circuitry processed the frequency-modulated signal to produce a voltage proportional to pressure.

The performance characteristics reported for the uncompensated Laurens unit were quite good. The sinusoidal frequency response was uniform from 0 to 100 Hz. Between this frequency and 5000 Hz, there are three resonant peaks, the largest of which occured at about 2.5 kHz. In subsequent studies, Allard (1962) reported that the frequency response was uniform from 0 to 1000 Hz.

The practicality and dependability of the catheter type strain gauge transducer undoubtedly led to efforts to use strain-gauge elements to create a catheter-tip pressure transducer. The first of such devices was described by Warnick and Drake (1958); this device, shown in Fig. 16, soon became available commercially (Statham, Oxnard, CA). The sensing-element was an expandable ridged metal sleeve mounted inside the tip of a catheter. Around the sleeve was wrapped the strain-gauge wire. The even solid lines represent the two active elements; the wavy lines represent the inactive elements used for temperature compensation only. Pressure applied to the lumen of the catheter expands the sleeve and stretches the two strain-sensitive wires, thereby producing a resistance change. The frequency response of the catheter-tip transducer extended to beyond 1000 Hz in fluid. With rated excitation (7.5 volts DC or AC rms), the sensitivity was on the order of 10 μV/mm Hg.

Angelakos (1964) took advantage of the fact that silicon exhibits a gauge factor ($\Delta R/R/\Delta L/L$), about 65 times that of the materials usually used in strain gauges, and constructed a catheter-tip pressure transducer in which a distensible diaphragm near the end of the catheter was coupled to four silicon bars. The arrangement was such that when pressure was applied to the diaphragm, two of the bars were stretched and two were compressed. All four strain-gauge elements were arranged in a bridge circuit, and temperature compensation was automatically obtained. He reported a natural frequency of 8 kHz, and a frequency response extending from 0 to 2 kHz. A range of 0–250 mm Hg, and a sensitivity of 200 μV/mm Hg were given. This device was commercially available for a time (Micro-Systems Inc., Pasadena, CA).

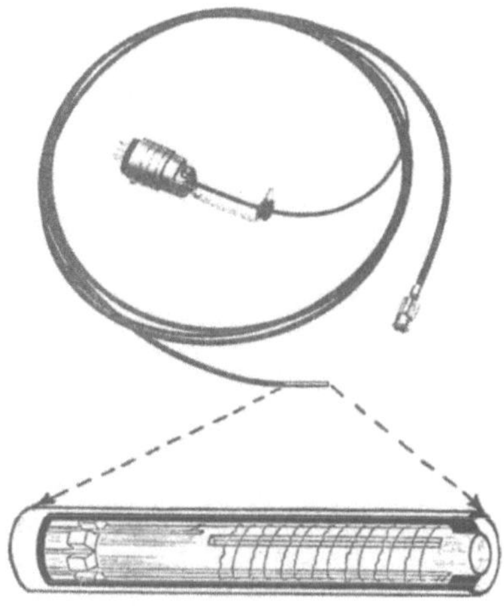

Fig. 16. Catheter-tip transducer with a hollow tip. (Redrawn from Warnick, A. and Drake, E. H., *IRE. Conv. Rec.* 1958, **Part 9,** 68–73.)

An interesting fiberoptic catheter-tip transducer was described by Clark et al. (1965). It consisted of a silvered mylar membrane (0.003 inch thick) mounted to the tip of 3 mm diameter catheter. The fiberoptic bundles were arranged coaxially in the catheter. The central bundle of about 200 glass fibers illuminated the center of the diaphragm. The light reflected from the diaphragm when deflected by pressure was carried up the outer bundle of glass fibers to a photodetector. An incandescent lamp illuminated the central fibers, and a photodiode was used to detect the reflected light. A frequency response from 0 to the audiofrequency range was reported.

The fiberoptic catheter-tip transducer described by Clark et al. has the potential to be disposable, because the catheter with its membrane and optical fibers are very inexpensive. The more expensive parts, the light source and photodetector, are permanent equipment. At present, several companies are investigating the potential of this technique to create an inexpensive disposable unit.

Although the Angelakos catheter-tip pressure transducer and its predecessors were available commercially, interest in such devices was limited; the reason is not known. In 1969, Millar started development of a rugged, easy-to-use catheter-tip pressure transducer in his home laboratory in Houston, TX. The first units (8F), one of which is shown in Fig. 17, had remarkably good performance characteristics, namely, a high output per mm Hg, and an extremely short response time (i.e., excellent high-frequency response). Millar and Baker (1973) presented the first paper describing the Millar

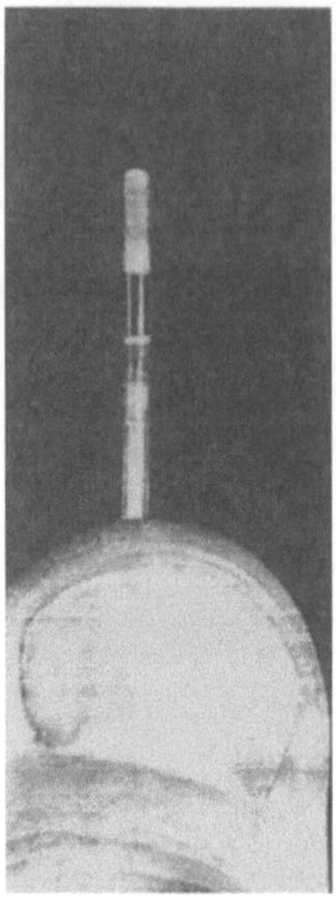

Fig. 17. The first Millar Mikro-Tip (8F) Teflon catheter transducer, held between the thumb and forefinger (catheter 1970). (Courtesy, Millar Instruments, Houston, TX.)

MIKRO-TIP catheter-tip pressure transducer that is the standard in the field today.

It is not difficult to foresee the direction to be taken by catheter-tip pressure transducers. Already, smaller units (e.g., 3F) are becoming available. Another evolutionary direction is the incorporation of flow sensors; this has already taken place. The next step is already at hand, namely, development of disposable units. Integrated-circuit fabrication techniques have made this possible, and several companies are now engaged in developing such prepackaged, sterilized, disposable transducers.

INDIRECT PRESSURE

Introduction

As stated previously, palpation of the arterial pulse dates from antiquity, and there developed special terms to describe its quality. For example, it exhibited frequency (pulsus frequens et rarus), magnitude (p. magnus et parvus), rate of dilation (p. celer et tardus), hardness or compressibility (p. durus et mollis), regularity or irregularity of rhythm (p. intermittens, alternans, intercurrens), and least, the form of the pulse wave (p. dicrotus seu bisferiens). These terms appear frequently in the medical literature. When graphic recording appeared in 1847, there arose the opportunity of recording the pulse and adding a quantitative meaning to these terms.

THE CONCEPT OF COUNTERPRESSURE

The first to record the human pulse was Vierordt (1855). A good description of his pulse recorder appeared in the March 1955 issue of the *Scientific American*. The report stated:

> "Professor Vierordt has been exhibiting a machine at Frankfort to record on paper the beatings of the pulse. The arm of the patient is placed in a longitudinal cradle and screwed down sufficiently to keep it steady. A small erection on one side holds a sort of lever worked on a hinge, at the end of which a pencil is inserted, the point of which has been dipped in Indian ink. The lever rests upon the pulse, and at every moment records the action."

The first high-fidelity pulse recorder was reported by Marey (1860), champion of the graphic method in physiology and medicine; his instrument is shown in Fig. 18. Close inspection of the record reveals the dicrotic notch. Having the ability to record the pulse waveform led naturally to a desire to quantitate its magnitude. In other words, how could it be used to measure blood pressure? The answer to this question took some time.

In a remarkable experiment, Marey (1876) found the way to use a graphic record of the pulse to determine blood pressure noninvasively. Marey's experiment introduced the concept of counterpressure; Fig. 19 illustrates the device employed by Marey. With the hand and forearm sealed in a water-filled compression chamber with a transparent window, the pressure therein was recorded on a smoked-drum kymograph (K). When the pressure in the chamber was increased by raising the water-filled reservoir (R), there appeared small-amplitude oscillations on the pressure record. As the pressure was raised continuously, the amplitude of the oscillations increased, reached a maximum, then decreased as shown. At a critical (suprasystolic) pressure, the forearm blanched.

The new information provided by Marey's experiment pertains to the counterpressure for blanching, and maximal oscillations. Marey knew that the point of blanching identified systolic pressure.

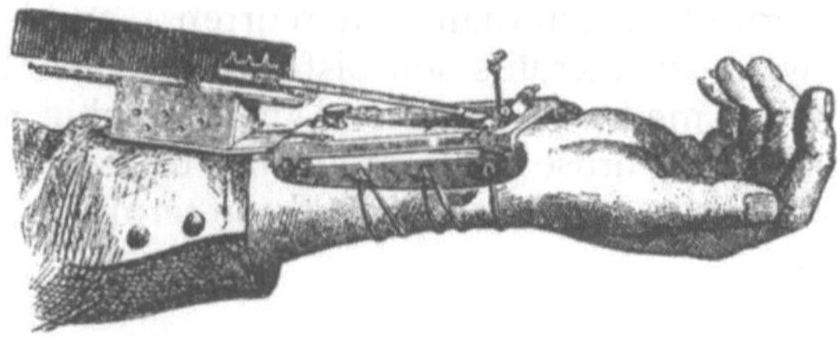

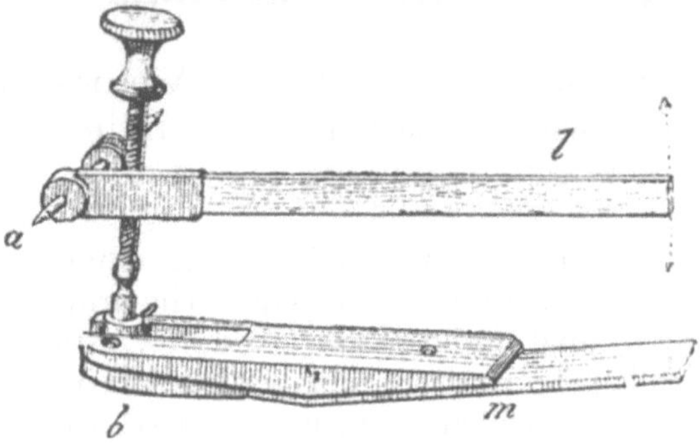

Fig. 18. Marey's pulse recorder (A) and adjustable lever in contact with the radial artery. (From Marey, E. J., 1860.)

Marey reasoned correctly that at the pressure for maximal oscillations, there is no tension on the arterial walls, and arterial pressure is freely communicated to the water in the chamber. Marey did not state that the counterpressure for maximal oscillations was equal to mean pressure. This fact was established much later by Posey et al. (1969). Nonetheless, Marey's experiment was the first to demonstrate what is now known as vascular unloading.

Obviously, Marey's water-filled plethysmograph was unsuitable for clinical use. Accordingly, Marey devised an air-filled instrument that applied counterpressure to a single digit, as shown in Fig. 20. The mercury manometer had a bore of one-third millimeter, and the finger was placed in a rubber sleeve within a rigid cylinder. A squeeze bulb was used to raise the counterpressure that was indicated by the mercury manometer. Unfortunately, the oscillations in the height of the mercury column were small owing to the use of air as the coupling medium. However, Marey noted that it required a very high counterpressure to make the oscillations disappear.

Mosso (1895) improved Marey's instrument so that all of the fingers were subjected to the counterpressure, as shown in Fig. 21A. A recording mercury manometer displayed the counterpressure and the oscillations. Figure 21B is a record obtained with

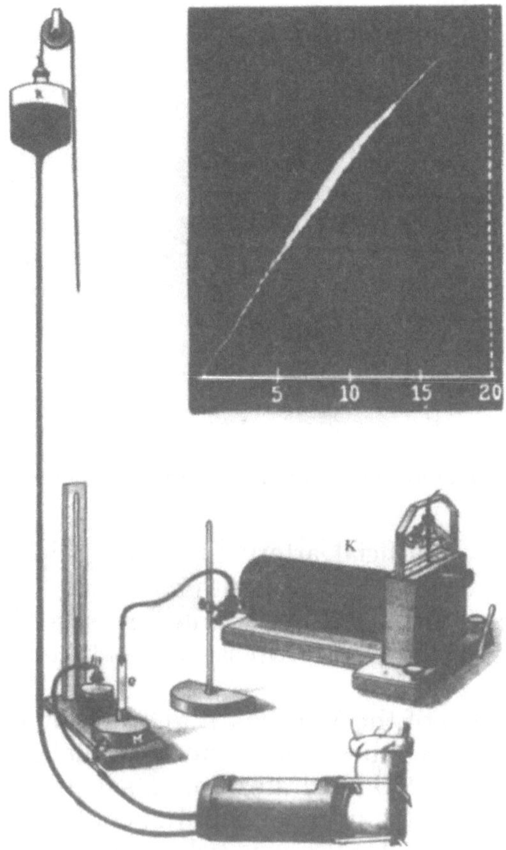

Fig. 19. Marey's arm-occluding method of measuring blood pressure. (From Marey, E. J., *Physiologie Experimentale*, Masson & Cie, Paris, 1876, vol. 2, pp. 317, 318.)

Mosso's instrument. The point of maximum oscillations was taken as diastolic pressure, and the point where they became very small was taken as systolic pressure. We now know that these criteria are incorrect. The paper that established the point of maximum oscillations as diastolic pressure was presented by Howell and Brush (1901), who based their conclusion on the amplitude of oscillations of a dog carotid artery in a compression chamber. A maximum-and-minimum reading mercury manometer (Fig. 8) was used to measure systolic and diastolic pressures in the contralateral carotid artery.

A different method of applying counterpressure was taken by Von Basch (1876), who employed a water-filled bag connected to a mercury manometer, as shown in Fig. 22A. The bag was placed on

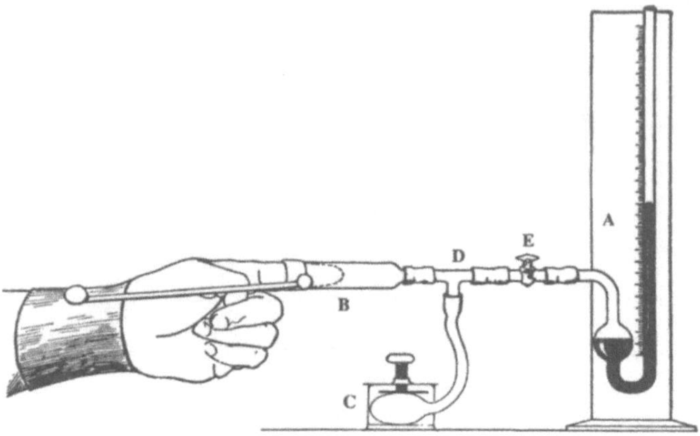

Fig. 20. Marey's method of using air to apply counterpressure to the digital arteries.

the skin over a superficial artery that was palpated distally. By pressing the bag against the skin with increased force, the mercury in the manometer displayed the counterpressure. When the distal pulse disappeared, the counterpressure was taken as systolic pressure.

Many versions of the Von Basch instrument appeared. Potain (1902) replaced the mercury manometer by a dial gauge; the system was air-filled. Figure 22B illustrates Potain's instrument. Potain also devised a small circular, air-filled bag that could be pressed against the skin when the distal pulse was palpated, as shown in Fig. 22C. All of these devices employed lateral counterpressure.

By the end of the 19th century, the concept of using a measured counterpressure to occlude blood flow in a superficial artery was well-established. The next step led directly to the modern methods of measuring blood pressure noninvasively. Almost simultaneously, Riva Rocci (1896) in Italy, and Hill and Barnard (1897) in England introduced the arm-encircling cuff to apply circumferential counterpressure to the brachial artery. Riva-Rocci's rubber cuff, that was 5 cm wide, is shown in Fig. 23A. Barnard and Hill's cuff, shown in Fig. 23B, consisted of a metal band under which was a narrow bladder that was inflated with a bicycle tire pump.

In a series of experiments, Von Recklinghausen (1901) showed that the newly introduced arm-encircling cuffs were too narrow, and gave a falsely high systolic pressure. To prove his point, Von Recklinghausen constructed wider cuffs, and measured pressure on one arm with them. Simultaneously, he used the 5 cm wide cuff on

A

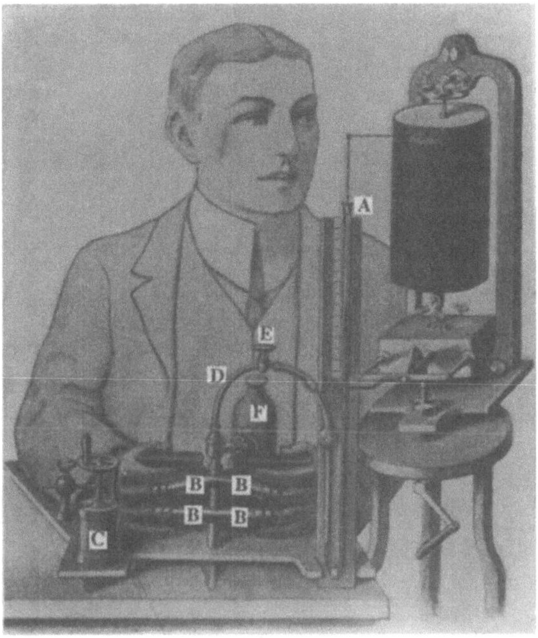

B

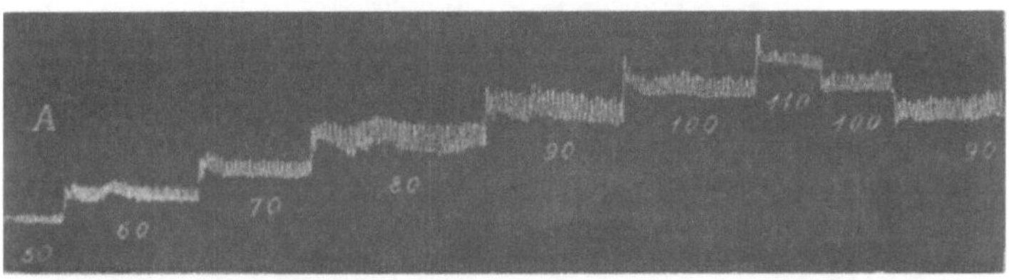

Fig. 21. Mosso's instrument for measuring blood pressure in the fingers (A), and a record obtained with it (B). (A, from *Arch. Ital. Biol.* 1895, **23**, 177; and B, from *Human Physiology* by L. Luciani, trans. by F. A. Wilby, 1911, MacMillan & Co., London.)

the other arm, using the palpatory method in both cases. He found that the 5 cm cuff produced pressures that were 15 to 20% higher than obtained with a 12 cm cuff.

The arm-encircling cuffs that provided circumferential counterpressure were used to determine systolic pressure with the palpatory method. Because it was often difficult to determine the appearance of the distal pulse during cuff deflation, Vaquez (1908) added a second, partially inflated, distal cuff, connected to a sensitive pressure indicator that facilitated detection of the appearance of the pulse. Figure 24 is an illustration of the Vaquez instrument that gained limited popularity.

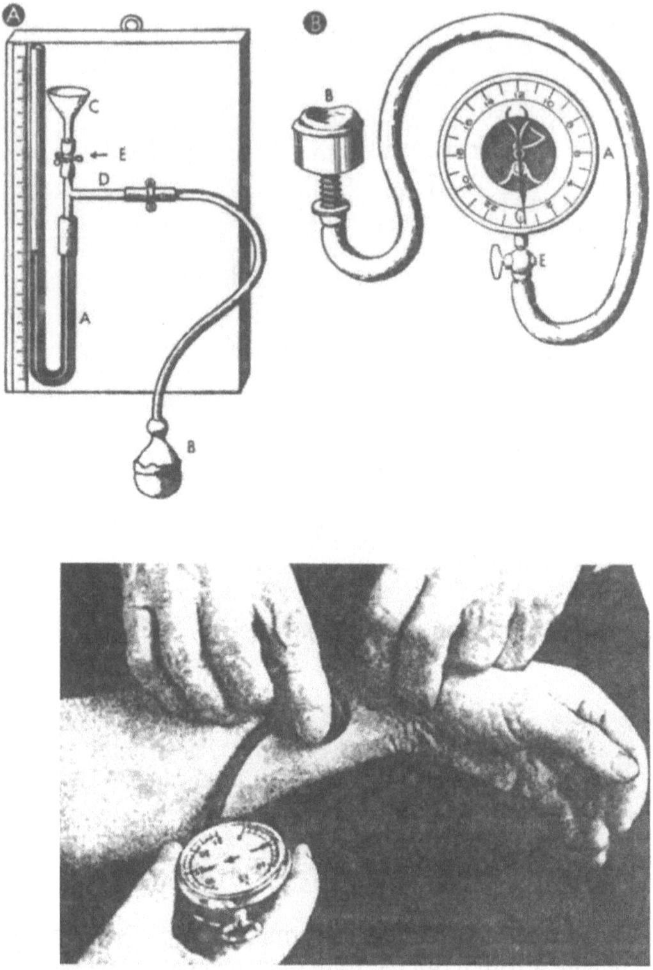

Fig. 22. Devices that employed lateral counterpressure to occlude a superficial artery. A, Von Basch (1876); B, Potain (1902); and C, Potain (1902).

Meanwhile, Erlanger (1904) described an instrument that resembled Mosso's, except that a Riva-Rocci cuff was used to apply the counterpressure. Figure 25A illustrates Erlanger's instrument that employed a mercury manometer to display cuff pressure, and a Marey sphygmoscope (B) to display cuff-pressure oscillations with a recording rambour (T). A sphygmoscope is an elastic balloon enclosed in a chamber connected to a sensitive recording tambour. The technique for displaying only cuff-pressure oscillations consisted of first allowing the tambour to be exposed to atmospheric pressure when a steady pressure was applied to the cuff causing the balloon

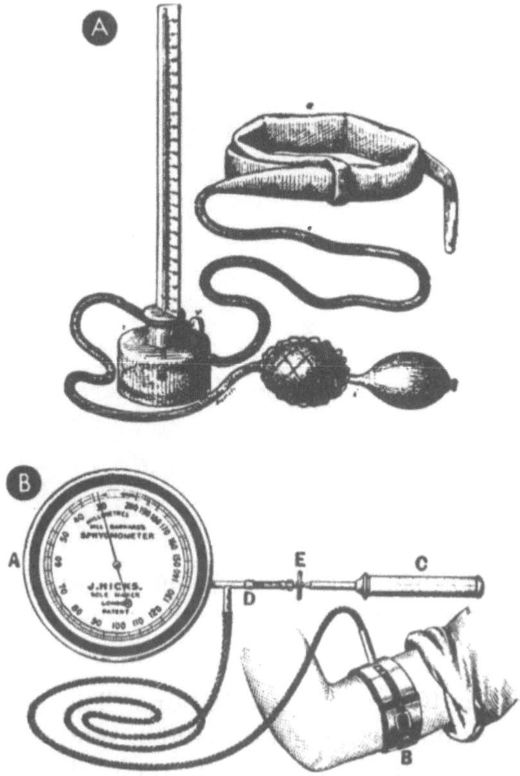

Fig. 23. The first arm-encircling arterial-occluding cuffs. A, Riva-Rocci's cuff (from Luciani, L., *Human Physiology*, trans. by F. A. Welby, Macmillan & Co., Ltd., London, 1911, vol. 1, 592 pp.). B, Hill and Barnard's cuff (from Hill, L. and Barnard, H., *Brit. M. J.* **2,** 904, 1897, with permission).

(B) to expand. Then, the mercury manometer was shut off from the cuff, and the tambour was switched to detect and display the small pressure oscillations in the chamber, owing to pulsation of the balloon. The procedure was repeated for different cuff pressures. Figure 25B illustrates one of Erlanger's records. Unfortunately, Erlanger did not know that the sphygmoscope was nonlinear, i.e., the same pulsatile pressure at a different level of counterpressure would not be displayed with the same amplitude. It is well to remember that Erlanger distinguished himself later by receiving the Nobel Prize with Gasser, for discovering the fundamental relationship between nerve conduction velocity and fiber diameter.

The major difficulties with the oscillometric method related to the need for graphic recording to identify the transitions in the

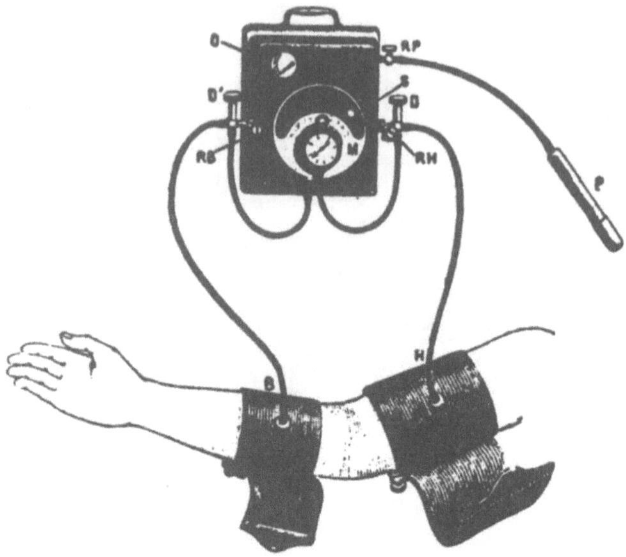

Fig. 24. Vaquez method of using a partially inflated distal cuff, connected to a sensitive pressure indicator, to identify appearance of the pulse during cuff deflation. (From Vaquez, 1908.)

amplitude of the cuff-pressure oscillations. The need for graphic recording was eliminated by Pachon (1909), who devised the dual-dial instrument shown in Fig. 26A. The circular dial gauge identified cuff pressure, and the sector gauge displayed cuff pressure oscillations only. An ingenious method was used to display cuff-pressure oscillations with constant sensitivity, regardless of the magnitude of the counterpressure. Figure 26B illustrates the method in which the outside of an aneroid gauge (C) was exposed only to the counterpressure acting on the cuff (B). This was accomplished by adjusting valve V so that only a small port transmitted the steady pressure to the circular dial gauge (M), and the outside of the aneroid (C). The inside of the aneroid was connected directly to the cuff (B) that was inflated by pump P. Thus, the outside of the aneroid was exposed to the cuff pressure, and the inside was exposed to the cuff pressure plus oscillations. Therefore, the pointer (l) of the aneroid displayed only cuff-pressure oscillations.

Apparently, elimination of graphic recording for displaying cuff pressure oscillations did not meet the needs of all, for Plesch (1931) revived it in an interesting way. In his instrument shown in Fig. 27A, movement of the graphic record tracked cuff pressure. The amplitude of cuff-pressure oscillations was displayed by an oscillometer operating on the principle used by Pachon. At a glance,

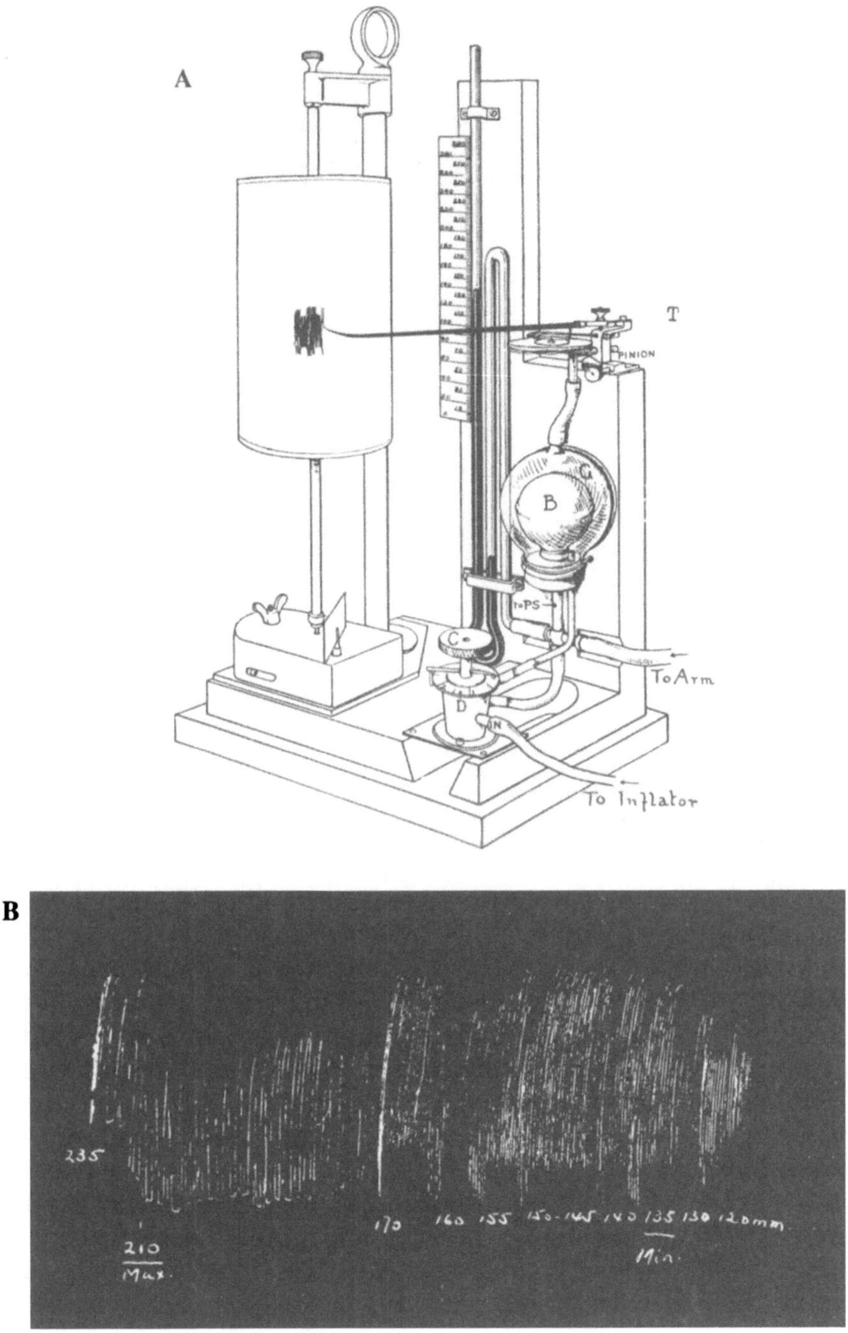

Fig. 25. Erlanger's oscillometric instrument (A) and a record obtained with it (B). (From Erlanger, J., 1904.)

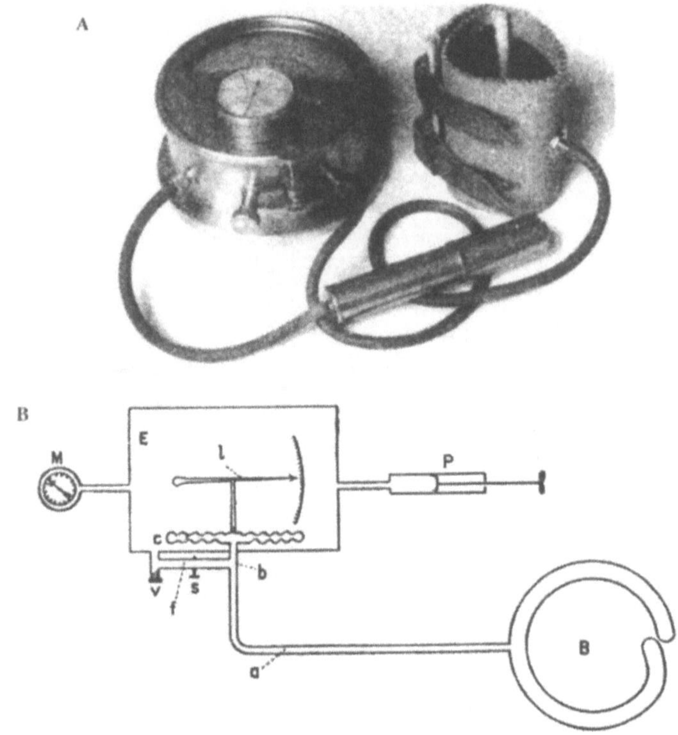

Fig. 26. Pachon's oscillometer, in which the circular dial gauge (M) identified cuff pressure, and the large sector gauge displayed cuff-pressure oscillations. (From Pachon, V., 1909.)

the transitions in the amplitude spectrum could be identified clearly (Fig. 27B).

What we now know as the flush method is an ingenious example of the application of counterpressure to obtain systolic pressure. Introduced in 1899 by Gaertner, the method employs an occluding cuff placed over the finger, that is first made anemic prior to inflating the cuff. Figure 28 illustrates the method in which the digit is first rendered bloodless by wrapping tightly with an elastic (Esmarch) bandage. Then, the cuff was applied, pressurized to well above suspected systolic pressure, and then the elastic bandage removed. When observing the counterpressure displayed by the mercury manometer, systolic pressure was read when the digit became flushed with blood.

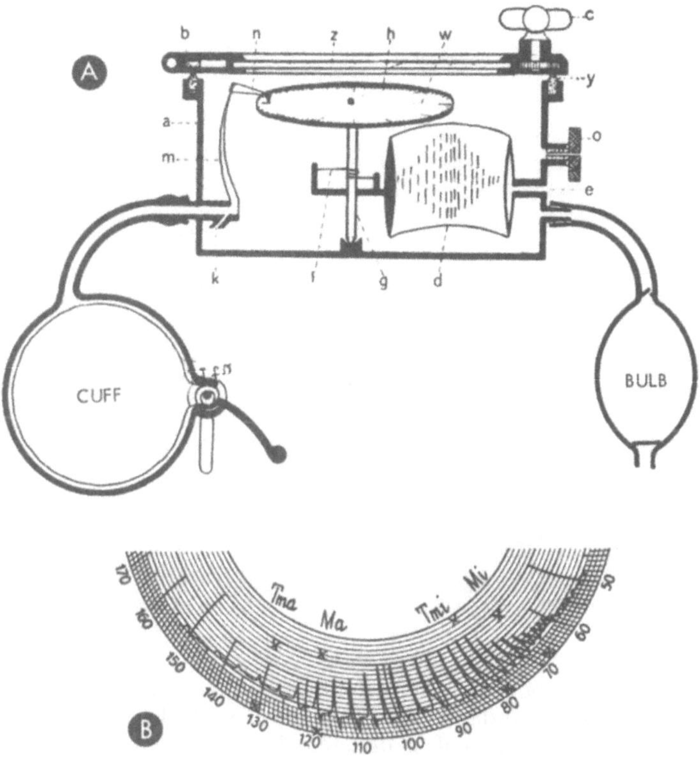

Fig. 27. Plesch's graphic recording oscillometer, in which the graphic record was caused to be moved by cuff pressure (From Plesch, 1931).

AUSCULTATORY METHOD

In his MD thesis, Korotkoff (1905) described a technique for evaluating the effectiveness of collateral circulation by compressing an artery and measuring blood pressure distally, using a Riva-Rocci (14″ long, 3–4″ wide) cuff. During deflation of the cuff, appearance of the pulse identified systolic pressure. Korotkoff wanted to be sure that blood flow had been arrested by the arterial compression, and believed that absence of the distal pulse was an unreliable indicator of the arrest of blood flow. He wrote (Segall, 1980):

> "Furthermore, if the volume of blood reaching the periphery through a partial occlusion is rather small, pulsations are not transmitted to

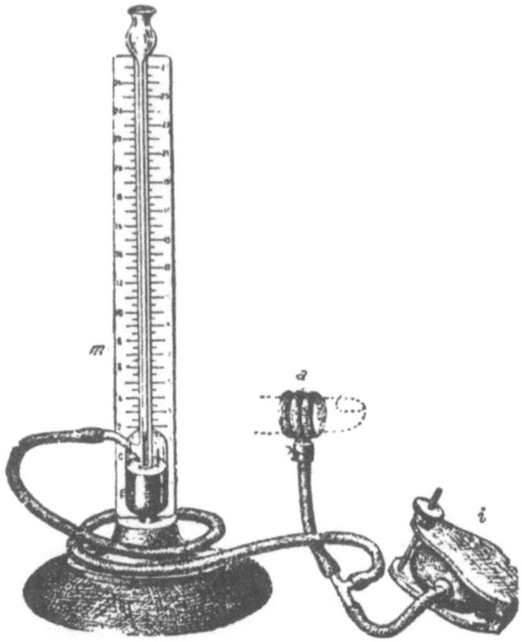

Fig. 28. The flush method introduced by Gaertner. The digit is first rendered anemic with an elastic bandage; then, the cuff is applied, and inflated. Then the bandage is removed and the cuff is deflated. The cuff pressure at which the digit became flushed, identified systolic pressure (From Gaertner, 1899).

the periphery; they may appear in the presence of a greater volume of blood flowing through collaterals, i.e. when in spite of compression of the main artery the lumen of the collaterals remain open. Thus, the absence of a pulsation within the periphery is not indicative of the fact that the artery is fully compressed. In this respect, our hearing is a better guide. I pointed out in my reports of Nov. 8th and Dec. 13th that immediately below a fully compressed artery (with complete occlusion of the lumen), no sound is heard. As soon as the first drops of blood escape from under the compressed site, we hear a clapping sound, very distinctly. This sound is heard, when the compressed artery is released, even before the appearance of pulsations in the peripheral branches. Hence, whenever I had to compress for complete occlusion of a vessel, I proceeded with auscultation of the artery immediately below (beyond) the compressed site in order to check the compression, and found the phonendoscope (stethoscope) extremely useful for this procedure."

From the foregoing, it is clear that Korotkoff measured blood pressure routinely with the palpatory method, and believed that appearance of the distal pulse was an insensitive indicator of systolic pressure. It is equally obvious that Korotkoff knew that partial occlusion of a vessel produced sound that ceased when blood flow was arrested. Therefore, it is very logical that he was led to develop the auscultatory method. In 1905, Korotkoff presented a short paper to the Imperial Military Medical Academy in St. Petersburg. Figure 29 is a copy of his paper, and the following is a translation by Badger (Geddes et al., 1966).

On the Subject of Methods of Determining Blood Pressure

(From the Clinic of Prof. S. P. Fedorov)

Dr. N. S. Korotkoff:

> "On the basis of his observations, this reporter has arrived at the conclusion that a completely compressed artery in a normal condition does not produce any sound. Taking advantage of this situation the reporter proposes the sound method for determining the blood pressure in humans. The sleeve (cuff) of Riva-Rocci is placed on the middle ⅓ of the arm toward the shoulder. The pressure in the sleeve is raised quickly until it stops the circulation of the blood beyond the sleeve. Thereupon, permitting the mercury manometer to drop, a child's stethoscope is used to listen to the artery directly beyond the sleeve. At first no audible sound is heard at all. As the mercury manometer falls to a certain height the first short tones appear, the appearance of which indicates the passage of part of the pulse wave under the sleeve. Consequently, the manometer reading at which the first tones appear corresponds to the maximum pressure. With a further fall of the mercury in the manometer systolic pressure murmurs are heard which change again to a sound (secondary). Finally, all sounds disappear. The time at which the sounds disappear indicates a free passage of the pulse wave; in other words, at the moment the sounds disappear, the minimum blood pressure in the artery exceeds the pressure of the sleeve. Consequently, the reading of the manometer at this time corresponds to the minimum blood pressure. Experiments on animals gave positive results. The first sound-tones appear (10–12 mm) sooner than the pulse, for the perception of which (r. art. radialis) the breakthrough of a greater part of the pulse wave is required."

Др. Н. С. Коротковъ. **Къ вопросу о методахъ изслѣдованія кровяного давленія (изъ клиники проф. С. П. Ѳедорова).**

На основаніи своихъ наблюденій докладчикъ пришелъ къ тому заключенію, что вполнѣ сжатая артерія при нормальныхъ условіяхъ не даетъ никакихъ звуковъ. Воспользовавшись этимъ явленіемъ онъ предлагаетъ звуковой методъ опредѣленія кровяного давленія на людяхъ. Рукавъ Rivva-Rocci накладывается на среднюю ⅓ плеча; давленіе въ рукавѣ быстро повышается до полнаго прекращенія кровообращенія ниже рукава. Затѣмъ, предоставивъ ртути манометра падать, дѣтскимъ стетоскопомъ выслушиваютъ артерію тотчасъ ниже рукава. Сперва не слышно никакихъ звуковъ. При паденіи ртути манометра до извѣстной высоты появляются первые короткіе тоны, появленіе которыхъ указываетъ на прохожденіе части пульсовой волны подъ рукавомъ. Слѣдов., цифры манометра, при которыхъ появился первый тонъ соотвѣтствуютъ максимальному давленію. При дальнѣйшемъ паденіи ртути въ манометрѣ слышатся систолическіе компрессіонные шумы, которые переходятъ снова въ тоны (вторые). Наконецъ, всѣ звуки исчезаютъ. Время исчезновенія звуковъ указываетъ на свободную проходимость пульсовой волны; другими словами, въ моментъ исчезанія звуковъ минимальное кровяное давленіе въ артеріи превысило давленіе въ рукавѣ. Слѣд., цифры манометра въ это время соотвѣтствуютъ минимальному кровяному давленію. Опыты на животныхъ дали положительные результаты. Первые звуки-тоны появляются (на 10—12 mm.) раньше, нежели пульсъ, для ощущенія котораго (r. av. radialis) требуется прорывъ большей части пульсовой волны.

Fig. 29. Korotkoff's paper on the auscultatory method. *Bull. Imp. Mil. Acad.*, St. Petersburg, 1905, **17**, 365–367.

Korotkoff's method was not embraced immediately in the English-speaking world, despite its simplicity and clinical applicability. Controversy continued on the systolic and diastolic criteria with the oscillometric method. To make matters worse, the pressures obtained with Korotkoff's method were compared to those obtained with the oscillometric method. At that time, there were few high-fidelity pressure-recording instruments that could be used to measure arterial pressure directly. The first American report on Korotkoff's method was presented by Gittings (1910), who wrote:

> "His (Korotkoff's) method has been thoroughly studied, especially in Germany and has been adopted by many observers as a routine procedure. Apparently, it has been little, if at all, discussed in the

> American and English literature, and in view of the importance of proving or disproving the claims that have been made for it, it has seemed advisable to present this preliminary report in the hope that others may be induced to gather testimony."

The first British report to acknowledge Korotkoff's discovery was presented four years later by MacWilliam and Melvin (1914). The first English report to compare auscultatory and directly measured pressure was by Warfield (1912), who used the anesthetized dog. A maximum/minimum-reading mercury manometer (Fig. 8) was used to measure systolic and diastolic pressures in the contralateral femoral artery. He found that the first sound agreed with directly measured systolic pressure. However, the point of muffling was found to correlate with diastolic pressure. It was not until 1932 that directly recorded pressures were compared with those obtained with the auscultatory method. Wolf and von Bonsdorff (1932) made such comparisons in conscious human subjects. They found that one-third of the auscultatory comparisons were within 5 mm Hg of directly measured pressure. It should be recognized that at that time, the importance of using the proper cuff width was not fully recognized. This came about when direct/indirect comparisons began to be made on children.

So characteristic was the nature of the sounds heard during cuff deflation that it prompted Goodman and Howell (1911) to divide it into five phases, based on the intensity of sounds. By measuring the intensity of the sounds in the papers by Groedel and Miller (1943), Korns (1926) and Rappaport and Luisada (1944), it is possible to compose a spectrogram that identifies the various phases, as shown in Fig. 30. This figure should be compared to Fig. 15 (Part 2), in which the acoustic energy is plotted for each Korotkoff sound complex heard during cuff deflation.

With the auscultatory method, the systolic pressure criterion is not in doubt. However, there is uncertainty about the diastolic end point. All the research to date has shown that in some subjects, silence is the best point; in others, it is the point of muffling. As shown in Fig. 15 (Part 2), the onset of the Korotkoff sounds and the distal pulse, both occur earlier and earlier in the cardiac cycle, with cuff deflation from above systolic pressure. Below diastolic pressure, there is no decrease in appearance time. To date, no use has been made of this fact to improve the accuracy of the diastolic criterion. It is hoped that a future history of this subject will recount such a use.

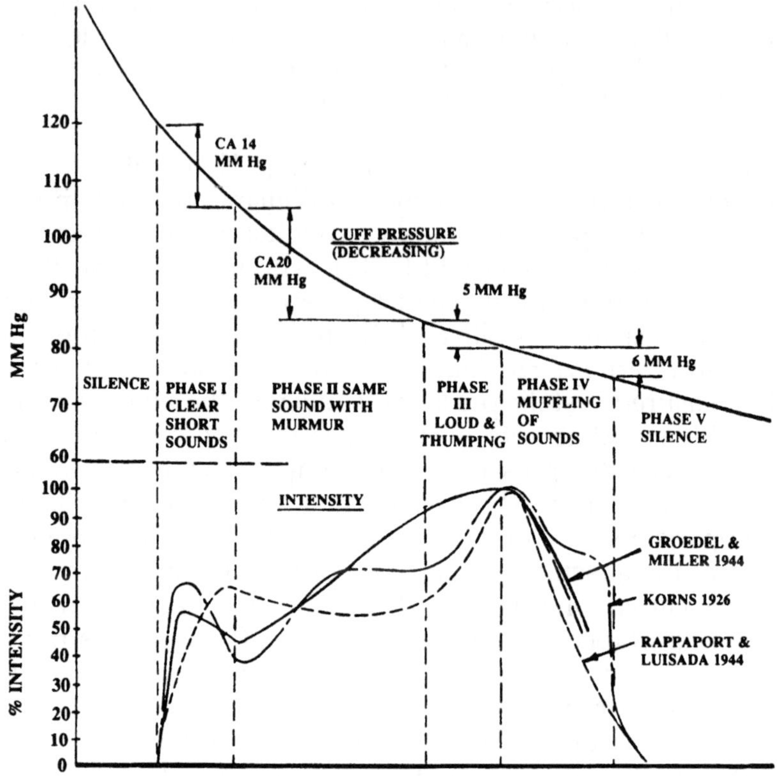

Fig. 30. Relative intensity of sounds during cuff deflation. (Composed from data in the papers by Goodman and Howell, 1911; Groedel and Miller, 1943; Korns, 1926; and Rappaport and Lusada, 1944.)

REFERENCES

Allard, E. M. Sound and pressure signals obtained from a single intracardiac transducer. IRE (IEEE) trans. *Bio-Med. Elect.* 1962, **BME9(2),** 74–77.

Angelakos, E. T. Semiconductor pressure microtransducers. *Amer. Journ. Med. Elect.* 1964, **3,** 266–270.

Broemser, P. Ein optisches Plattenmanometer. *Zeits. fur Biol.* 1927, **86,** 619–625.

Clark, F. J., Schmidt, E. M., and DeLaCroix, R. F. Fiber optic blood pressure catheter with frequency response from DC into the audio range. *Proc. Natl. Electronics Conf.* 1965, **21,** 213–215.

Einthoven, W. Ein neues Galvanometer. *Ann. Phys.* 1903, **12 Suppl. 4,** 1059–1071.

Erlanger, J. A new instrument for determining the minimum and maximum blood-pressures in man. *Johns Hopkins Hosp. Rep.* **12,** 53–110, 1903, 1904.

Fick, A. Ein neuer Blutwellenzeichner. Reicherts u. du Bois Reymond's *Arch. Anat Physiol.* 1864, **S583,** 543–548.

Fick, A. Ein verbessung des Blutwellenzeichners Arch. f.d. ges. *Physiol.* 1883, 30, **S592,** 608–613.

Frank, O. Ein neves optisches Federmanometer. *Zeits. f. Biol.* 1924, **82,** 49–65.

Frank, O. Kritik der elastesctuchen Manometer. *Zeits. f. Biol.* 1903, **49,** 445–613.

Gaertner, G. Uber einen neuen Blutdruckmesser. *Wein Klin. Wchnschr.* 1899, **49,** 1412–1418.

Garten, S. Beitrage zur Lehre vom Kreislauf. *Zeits. f. Biol.* 1916, **66,** 23–82.

Gauer, O. H. and Gienapp, E. A miniature pressure-recording device. *Science* 1950, **112,** 404–405.

Geddes, L. A. and Bourland, J. D. Estimation of the damping coefficient of damped and underdamped resonant frequencies of catheter–transducer pressure-measuring systems. *Journ. Clin. Eng.* 1988, **13(1),** 59–62.

Geddes, L. A. and Hoff, H. E. The capillary electrometer. *Arch. Internationales d'Histoire des Sciences.* 1961, (July–Dec.), **56, 57,** 275–290.

Geddes, L. A., Hoff, H. E., and Badger, A. S. Introduction of the auscultatory method of measuring blood pressure—including a translation of Korotkoff's original paper. *Cardiovascular Research Center Bull.* 1966, **5(2),** 57–74.

Gilson, W. E. Photoelectric manometer, improved design. *Electronics* 1943, **16,** 112, 140.

Gittings, J. C. Auscultatory blood-pressure determinations. *Arch. Int. Med.* 1910, **6,** 196–204.

Golz, G. and Gaule, J. Ueber die Druckverhaltnisse im Innen des Herzens. *Arch. ges. Physiol. des Menschen u.d. Thieren.* Bonn, 1878, **18,** 100–135.

Goodman, E. H. and Howell, A. A. Further clinical studies in auscultatory method of determining blood pressure. *Amer. Journ. Med. Sci.* 1911, **142,** 334–352.

Groedel, F. and Miller, M. Graphic study of auscultatory pressure measurement. *Exp. Med. Surg.* 1943, **1(2),** 148–162.

Grunbaum, O. F. F. On a new method of recording alterations of pressure. *Journ. Physiol.* 1897, 1898, **22,** XLIX-LI.

Grundfest, H. and Hay, J. J. A strain-gauge recorder for physiological volume, pressure, and deformation measurement. *Science* 1945, **101,** 255, 256.

Hales, S. Statical Essays Haemostaticks vol. 2, 3rd Ed., W. Innys and R. Marby, eds., London, 1738, 361 pp.

Hales, S. Statical Essays *Vegetable Stabicks,* vol. 1, 3rd Ed., 1738, W. Innys and R. Marby, London, 1738, 376 pp.

Hamilton, W. F., Brewer, G., and Brotman, I. Pressure pulse contours in the intact animal. *Amer. Journ. Physiol.* 1934, **107,** 427–435.

Harvey, W. Exercitatio Anatomica de Motu Cordis et Sangiunis in Animalibus. English trans. by Leake, C. D. Chas. C. Thomas, Springfield, IL. 1931, 150 pp.

Hill, L. and Barnard, H. A simple and accurate form of sphygmometer or arterial pressure gauge contrived for clinical use. *Brit. Med. Journ.* 1897, **2,** 904.

Hoff, H. E., Geddes, L. A., and Guillemin, R. The anemograph of Onsen-Bray. *Hist. Med. Allied Sev.* 1957, **12(4),** 424–448.

Howell, W. H. and Brush, C. E. A critical note upon clinical methods of measuring blood pressure. *Boston Med. & Surg. Journ.* 1901, **145,** 146–151.

Hurthle, K. Beitrage zur Hamodynamik. *Archiv. f. d. ges. Physiol.* 1890, **47,** 1–47.

Korns, H. M. The nature and time relations of the compression sounds of Korotkoff in man. *Amer. Journ. Physiol.* 1926, **76,** 247–264.

Korotkoff, N. S. On the subject of methods of measuring blood pressure. *Bull. Imp. Military Med. Acad.* St. Petersburg, 1905, **11,** 365–367.

Korotkoff, N. S. Experiments for Determining the Efficiency of Arterial Collaterals. M.D. Thesis, trans. by H. N. Segall. Limited Publication. Montreal, 1980, Mansfield Book Mart.

Kubicek, W., Sedgwick, F. P., and Visscher, M. B. Adaptation of the glass spoon manometer to physiological studies. *Rev. Sci. Instrs.* 1941, **12,** 101, 102.

Lambert, E. H. and Wood, E. H. The use of a resistance wire, strain-gauge manometer to measure intraarterial pressure. *Proc. Soc. Exp. Biol. Med.* 1947, **64,** 186–190.

Landois, *see* Luciani, L. *Human Physiology.* trans. by F. A. Welby, Mac-Millan Co., London, 1911, vol. 1, 592 pp.

Laurens, P., Bouchard, F., Brial, E., Cornu, C., Baculard, P., and Soulie, P. Bruits et pressions cardiovasculaires. *Arch. Mal. de Coeur* 1959, **52,** 121–132.

Ludwig, C. Beitrage zur kenntniss des Einfluisses der Respirations bewegungen auf den Blutlauf im Aortensysteme. *Mullers Archiv. Anat.* 1847, pp. 240–302.

MacWilliam, J. A. and Melvin, G. S. Systolic and diastolic blood pressure criteria with special reference to the auscultatory method. *Brit. Med. Journ.* 1914, **1,** 693–697.

Marey, E. J. Recherches sur l'etat de la circulation d'appes les caracteres du pouls fournis par les nouveaux sphygmographe. *Journ. Physiol. de l'Hommie et Animaux* 1860, **3,** 241–274.

Marey, E. J. Physiologie Experimentale. Paris, 1876. Masson & Cie, 388 pp.

Marey, E. J. La Circulation du Sang. G. Masson, Paris, 1881, 745 pp.

Millar, H. D. and Baker, L. E. A stable ultraminiature transducer. *Med. Biol. Eng. Comput.* 1973, **11(1),** 86–89.

Mosso, A. Sphygmomanometre pour mesurer le pression du sang chez l'homme. *Arch. Ital. Biol.* 1895, **23,** 177–197.

Pachon, V. Oscillometre sphygmomanometrique a grande sensibilite constante. *Comptes Rendus Soc. Biol.* 1909, **66,** 776–779.

Peimme, T. E. Pressure measurement: electrical pressure transducers. *Prog. Cardiovasc. Dis.* 1963, **5(6),** 574–594.
Plesch, J. Tonoszillographie und Blutdruckkurve. *Med. Klin.* 1931, **27,** 1557.
Poiseuille, J. L. M. La Force du Coeur Aortique. Thesis presented to the Faculty of Medicine, Univ. Paris Aug. 8, 1828. Paris, 1828, Didiot le Jeune.
Posey, J. A., Geddes, L. A., Williams, H., and Moore, A. G. The meaning of the point of maximum oscillations in cuff pressure in the indirect measurement of blood pressure. Part 1. *Cardiovascular Res. Cent. Bull.* 1969, **8(1),** 15–25.
Potain, C. La measure de la pression arterielle chez l'homme. *Archiv. Physiol.* 1889, **50(1),** 558–569.
Potain, C. La Pression Arterielle. Masson & Cie, Paris 1902. 191 pp.
Rappaport, M. B. and Luisada, A. Indirect sphygmomanometry. *Journ. Lab. Clin. Med.* 1944, **29,** 638–656.
Rein, H. Photoelektrisches Transmissions-Manometer. *Arch. f.d.ges. Physiol.* 1940, **243,** 329–335.
Riva-Rocci, S. Un nuovo sfigmomanometro. *Gaz. Med. Torino* 1896, **47,** 981–996.
Schutz, E. Konstruktion einer manometrischen Sonde mit eletchrischer transmission. *Zeits. f. Biol.* 1931, **91,** 516–521.
Schutz, E. Demonstration eines neuen Blutdruckschreiber. *Klin. Wchnschv.* 1937, **10,** 11–37.
Segall, H. N. (Korotkoff's thesis). Experiments for determining the efficiency of arterial collaterals. N. S. Korotkoff. Mansfield, Montreal, Canada, 1980, Ltd. ed. of 250 copies.
Simmonds, E. E. 1942, US Patent 2,292,549.
Tomlinson, H. On the increase in resistance to the passage of an electric current produced by stretching. *Proc. Royal Soc.* (London) 1876, 1877, **25,** 451–453.
Vaquez, H. Sphygmo-signal. *Comptes Rendus Soc. Biol.* 1908, **1,** 875–877.
Vierordt, K. Die lehre von Arterienpuls. Braunshweig
Von Recklinghausen, H. Uber Blutdruckmessung beim Menschen. *Arch. exp. Path. Pharmakol.* 1901, **46,** 78–132.
Wagner, R. Die Beeinflussung des Druckablautes. *Zeits. f. Biol.* 1932, **92,** 54–85.
Warfield, L. M. Studies in auscultatory blood pressure phenomena. *Arch. Int. Med.* 1912, **10,** 258–267.
Warnick, A. and Drake, E. H. A new intracardiac pressure measuring system for infants and adults. *IRE Convention Rec.* 1958, **Part 9,** 68–73.
Wetterer, E. Einl neue manometrische Sonde mit elektischer Transmission. *Zeits. f. Biol.* 1943, **101,** 332–350.
Wiggers, C. J. and Baker, W. R. A new universal optical manometer. *Journ. Lab. Clin. Med.* 1924, **10,** 54–56.
Wiggers, C. J. Some factors contributing to the shape of the pressure curve in the right ventricle. *Amer. Journ. Physiol.* 1914, **33,** 382–396.
Wolff, H. J. and Von Bonsdorff, B. Blutige Messung der absoluten Sphygmograms beim Menschen. *Zeits. Exp. Med.* 1931, **79,** 569–577.

Index

D

E

F

G

H

I

K

MIX
Papier aus verantwortungsvollen Quellen
Paper from responsible sources
FSC® C105338

If you have any concerns about our products,
you can contact us on
ProductSafety@springernature.com

In case Publisher is established outside the EU,
the EU authorized representative is:
Springer Nature Customer Service Center GmbH
Europaplatz 3, 69115 Heidelberg, Germany

Printed by Libri Plureos GmbH
in Hamburg, Germany